# CARNIVORE: WHAT, WHY, HOW

## THE WISDOM OF PRACTICING CARNIVORES

ZHAMEESHA LLC
ATLANTIS, FL (USA)

# Carnivore : What, Why, How

## The Wisdom of Practicing Carnivores

### Copyright © 2024 by Stuart Barry Malin

ISBN 978-1-951645-24-3
First Edition, Print on Demand
Released 2025-12-18
Most recently updated 2026-02-20

Published by Zhameesha LLC
Atlantis, Florida USA
https://www.zhameesha.com

This book is a work of enthusiasm.

BISAC Subject Headings (www.bisg.org)
HEA048000   HEALTH & FITNESS / Diet & Nutrition / General
SEL000000   SELF-HELP / General
POL000000   POLITICAL SCIENCE / General

12 11 10 9 8 7 6 5 4 3 2 1

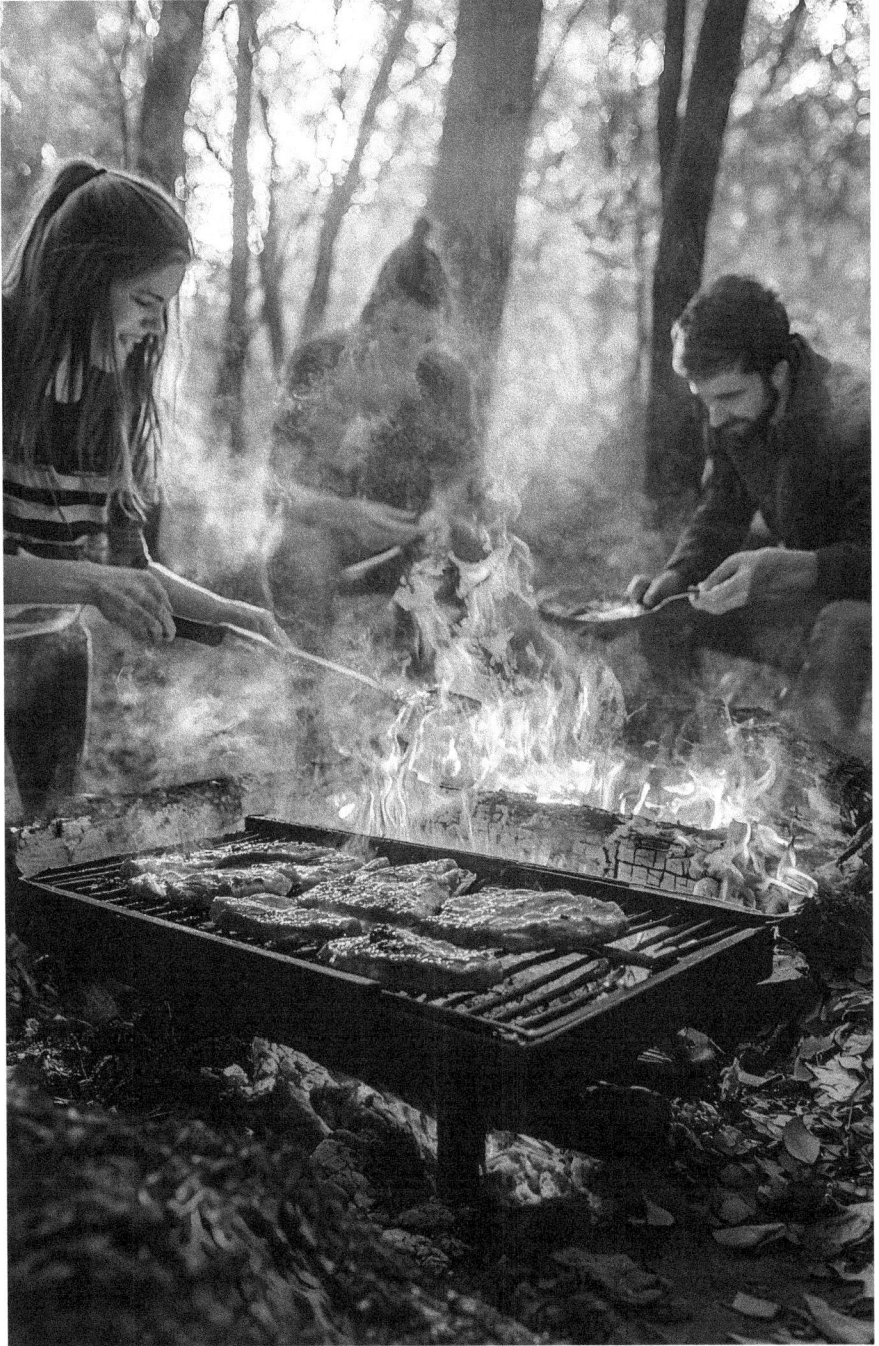

Carnivore: What, Why, How

**W**elcome to **Carnivore: What, Why, How**, a thought-provoking journey that will challenge your beliefs, spark new ideas, and transform your perspectives. In these pages, you'll explore an array of sources that provide a multifaceted view of the carnivore lifestyle, extending beyond its dietary restrictions to encompass a distinct approach to health, social interactions, and personal identity.

Overall, the sources present a portrait of the carnivore lifestyle as a multifaceted approach to health and well-being that extends beyond dietary choices. It involves a deep commitment to an animal-based diet, an active engagement in addressing social challenges and misinformation, and a willingness to embrace a way of eating that often runs counter to conventional dietary advice.

## About this Book

**This book represents the ideas of others**

The content os this book is derived from "Sources" — YouTube videos that are publicly available (or were at the time of the production).

- The statements made in the source material are best considered the positions, beliefs, and assertions of the speakers.
- The YouTube videos were selected by Stuart, the editor.

The sources are all biased in favor of a meat-based diet and many argue compellingly against the consumption of plant-based foods.

**This book was produced using AI**

For this book, Stuart worked with Google's Gemini, in the context of NotebookLM.

- The YouTube videos were summarized and analyzed by the AI.
- The text sections include here were generated by the AI.
- Stuart engaged in conversations with the AI to explore the material offered by the sources. These are represented herein as well.

The AI is not infallible and may may mistakes or "hallucinate." Stuart has read all the generated content and edited for presentation quality and his best sense of accuracy.

## About the Sources

### Challenging Conventional Nutritional Wisdom

The sources often position the carnivore diet as a rejection of conventional nutritional wisdom, which they argue is based on flawed science and influenced by vested interests, such as the sugar industry and plant-based food companies. They encourage individuals to question established dietary guidelines and to explore alternative approaches that align with their personal experiences and beliefs.

### A Note on the Sources

It's important to recognize that the sources largely present a pro-carnivore perspective and may not fully represent the broader scientific consensus on these dietary approaches. Further research is needed to fully understand the long-term health implications of specific diets. It is always advisable to consult with a qualified healthcare professional before making any significant dietary changes.

## Disclaimer and a call for caution

The sources present a compelling, albeit preliminary, case for the potential benefits of a carnivore diet. They highlight its potential for reducing inflammation, improving metabolic health, and optimizing nutrient intake. However, they also emphasize the importance of individualization, mindful attention to potential nutrient deficiencies, and a gradual approach to adaptation.

> *It is essential to note that the information presented in these sources is primarily anecdotal and based on personal experiences and observations.*

More rigorous scientific research is needed to fully understand the long-term effects and potential risks and benefits of a carnivore diet.

> *The information presented here is based on the provided sources and should not be considered medical advice. Consulting with qualified healthcare professionals is crucial for personalized guidance.*

## Consult with your Physician

*It is important to consult with a healthcare professional before making any significant dietary changes, especially if you have pre-existing health conditions or are taking medications. The information presented here should not be considered medical advice.*

## How best to engage the content

You can peruse this book in any order that strikes you, including opening randomly, for, as you will find explored in various arenas and on some of the pages, the notion of "entanglement" is a compelling counter-argument to truly random

I (Stuart, the editor) once asked Pi (an AI collaborator of mine), "Can you explain 'entanglement' in a spiritual sense."
Here is what Pi replied with:

> In a spiritual sense, entanglement refers to the idea that everything in the universe, including living beings, is connected on a deeper, invisible level. This concept goes beyond the physical connections we can observe and suggests that there is an underlying unity that binds all things together.
>
> Entanglement in a spiritual context implies that our thoughts, emotions, and actions can influence and be influenced by the world around us in ways that might not be immediately obvious. It's often associated with ideas like synchronicity, karma, and the interconnectedness of all living things.
>
> The notion of spiritual entanglement encourages us to consider the impact of our choices on the world and on others, and to recognize that we are all part of a larger, interconnected whole.

> **Death is not an option, but Life is.**

If you don't choose Life,

You'll get a laborious ride to death,

Which will come perhaps as a welcomed exit.

> *To choose Carnivore is to choose Life.*

## Publisher's Note (February 2026)

When this book was first written, it stood on its own—an honest record of inquiry, experience, and understanding at a particular moment in time.

Since then, additional books have emerged from the same lived investigation into animal-based nutrition. Taken together, they now form what the author has come to recognize as **The Carnivore Continuum**: an evolving, experience-driven exploration of carnivore eating as it is actually practiced, questioned, challenged, and integrated over time.

This volume represents one position along that continuum. It reflects what was known, tested, and understood when it was written—and remains unchanged for that reason. Readers may encounter perspectives elsewhere in the series that refine, complicate, or extend what appears here. That is intentional.

The Continuum is not a doctrine.
It is a record of attention.

# Contents

## Chapter 5 — Adopting

## Chapter 6 — Plant

# Chapter 7 — Seed Oils

# Chapter 8 — Science

# The Sources

## Postmatter

# CHAPTER 1

# INTRODUCTION

## Key Aspects of the Carnivore Lifestyle

**Dietary Commitment:** The foundation of the carnivore lifestyle is a strict adherence to a diet consisting solely of animal products, primarily meat, eggs, and seafood. This commitment involves eliminating all plant-based foods, including fruits, vegetables, grains, and even honey. The sources emphasize the importance of choosing high-quality, nutrient-dense animal products, such as fatty cuts of meat, pastured eggs, and wild-caught seafood.

**Health Transformation:** The sources, particularly those featuring medical professionals and individuals who have adopted a carnivore diet, present a compelling case for its potential health benefits. They highlight improvements in various health markers, including blood pressure, blood sugar levels, cholesterol, and inflammatory markers. Many sources suggest that a carnivore diet can help reverse metabolic dysfunction, manage autoimmune conditions, and improve mental well-being.

**Social Adaptation:** The sources acknowledge that the carnivore lifestyle often requires navigating social situations where dietary choices may be questioned or criticized. They offer practical tips for managing these interactions, such as bringing carnivore-friendly foods to gatherings or politely inquiring about food preparation methods at restaurants. Some sources also emphasize the importance of connecting with other carnivores through online communities or in-person meetups to find support, share experiences, and foster a sense of belonging.

**Philosophical Underpinnings:** The sources suggest that the carnivore lifestyle is often rooted in a deep conviction about the evolutionary appropriateness of an animal-based diet for humans. They cite anthropological evidence, historical accounts, and the physiological characteristics of the human digestive system to support the notion that humans are biologically adapted to thrive on a diet primarily composed of meat.

**Addressing Criticism and Misinformation:** Many sources, particularly those featuring medical professionals and experienced carnivores, actively challenge the mainstream narrative that demonizes saturated fat and cholesterol and promotes plant-based diets as superior for health. They cite scientific studies and personal experiences to counter these claims and advocate for a more nuanced understanding of human nutrition.

Carnivore: What, Why, How

## Challenges and Considerations

**Social Stigma and Misunderstandings:** The sources acknowledge that the carnivore lifestyle can be met with skepticism, criticism, and even hostility from family, friends, and healthcare professionals who adhere to conventional dietary guidelines. This social stigma can lead to feelings of isolation, judgment, and a sense of being misunderstood.

**Potential Nutrient Deficiencies:** The sources, while emphasizing the nutrient density of animal foods, also caution against potential nutrient deficiencies that might arise from a strict carnivore diet, particularly if organ meats are not included.

**Adaptation Period and Potential Side Effects:** The sources note that transitioning to a carnivore diet can involve an adaptation period during which individuals may experience side effects such as digestive disturbances, changes in bowel movements, and intense cravings for previously consumed foods.

## The Potential Benefits of the Carnivore Diet: Insights from the Sources

The sources offer a variety of perspectives on the potential benefits of a carnivore diet, primarily through the voices of medical professionals and individuals who have adopted this way of eating. While acknowledging the lack of long-term, large-scale studies, the sources highlight several areas where a carnivore diet might offer advantages:

### 1. Reducing Oxidative Stress and Inflammation

**Eliminating Vegetable Oils:** A central theme across the sources is the detrimental impact of vegetable oils on health, primarily due to their high concentration of polyunsaturated fatty acids (PUFAs) that are prone to oxidation. As discussed in our previous conversations, oxidized PUFAs contribute to oxidative stress, inflammation, and cellular damage. By eliminating vegetable oils, a carnivore diet removes a major source of these harmful compounds.

**Focusing on Nutrient-Dense Animal Foods:** The sources emphasize that animal-based foods are rich in nutrients that support the body's natural antioxidant defenses, including vitamins A, D, E, and K, as well as selenium and zinc. These nutrients play crucial roles in protecting cells from oxidative damage and reducing inflammation.

### 2. Addressing Chronic Health Conditions

**Reversing Metabolic Dysfunction:** Many sources, particularly those featuring medical professionals, point to the carnivore diet's potential for reversing metabolic dysfunction, including type 2 diabetes, insulin resistance, and obesity. They attribute this potential to the elimination of carbohydrates and the focus on animal fats, which promote stable blood sugar levels, reduce insulin spikes, and encourage the body to utilize fat for fuel.

**Improving Autoimmune Conditions:** Some sources suggest that a carnivore diet might benefit individuals with autoimmune conditions by reducing inflammation, improving gut health, and potentially addressing underlying food sensitivities that contribute to immune system dysregulation.

**Addressing Mental Health Concerns:** A few sources, including a medical professional, observe a connection between a carnivore diet and improvements in mental health, including reduced depression and anxiety.

### 3. Optimizing Nutrient Intake

**Bioavailability and Nutrient Density:** The sources highlight the superior bioavailability of nutrients found in animal-based foods compared to plant-based sources. This means that the body can more easily absorb and utilize nutrients from animal products.

**Meeting Specific Nutritional Needs:** Sources discussing the experiences of ex-vegans who transitioned to a carnivore diet emphasize the importance of addressing potential nutrient deficiencies, particularly those related to vitamin B12, iron, and zinc.

### 4. Simplifying Food Choices and Promoting Satiety

**Eliminating Processed Foods**: The restrictive nature of a carnivore diet naturally eliminates highly processed foods, which are often laden with added sugars, refined grains, and unhealthy fats. This simplification of food choices can reduce exposure to potential triggers for cravings, overeating, and metabolic disturbances.

**Promoting Satiety and Reducing Hunger:** The sources, including testimonials from individuals on a carnivore diet, suggest that the high protein and fat content of this way of eating promotes feelings of fullness and reduces hunger cravings.

## 5. Supporting Gut Health

**Eliminating Potential Irritants:** The sources, particularly those discussing digestive issues, suggest that a carnivore diet might benefit individuals with gut problems by eliminating potential irritants, such as fiber, lectins, and other plant compounds that can be difficult to digest.

**Promoting a Healthy Gut Microbiome:** Some sources suggest that a carnivore diet might support a healthy balance of gut bacteria, potentially by reducing the diversity of microbes and favoring those that thrive on animal-based substrates.

### Important Considerations

**Individual Variability:** The sources acknowledge that individual responses to a carnivore diet can vary significantly. Factors such as genetics, health history, gut microbiome composition, and nutrient status can influence how an individual's body responds to this way of eating.

**Potential Nutrient Deficiencies:** While emphasizing the nutrient density of animal foods, the sources also caution against potential nutrient deficiencies that might arise from a strict carnivore diet. They particularly highlight the importance of consuming organ meats to ensure adequate intake of nutrients like copper, vitamin A, and folate.

**Electrolyte Balance and Hydration:** The sources stress the importance of maintaining electrolyte balance and adequate hydration on a carnivore diet. They advise consuming sufficient sodium, potassium, and magnesium, which can be achieved through dietary sources and/or supplementation.

**Social and Practical Considerations:** The sources acknowledge the social challenges and potential inconvenience of adhering to a strict carnivore diet, particularly in settings where food choices are limited or social gatherings revolve around meals that include plant-based foods.

**Long-Term Sustainability and Adaptation:** The sources, particularly those featuring medical professionals, recommend a gradual transition to a carnivore diet to allow the body to adapt metabolically and minimize potential side effects, such as digestive disturbances.

## Understanding the Carnivore Diet:
## What You Gain from These Sources

Reading this collection of materials provides a comprehensive understanding of the carnivore diet from multiple angles. The sources move beyond simply listing potential benefits and instead explore the nuances of this lifestyle through scientific explanations, personal anecdotes, and the perspectives of both medical professionals and individuals who have embraced a carnivore way of eating.

Here's how these sources enhance your understanding:

**Challenging Conventional Dietary Thinking:** The sources directly confront the mainstream narrative that demonizes saturated fat and cholesterol while promoting plant-based diets as inherently healthier. They provide counter-arguments based on scientific studies and the experiences of individuals who have thrived on a carnivore diet.

**Deep Dive into Biological Mechanisms:** You'll gain insights into the biological mechanisms underlying the potential benefits of a carnivore diet. The sources explain concepts like oxidative stress, the role of PUFAs in inflammation, the impact of carbohydrates on blood sugar regulation, and the potential for nutrient deficiencies on a restricted diet.

**Addressing the Social and Emotional Aspects:** The sources acknowledge the social challenges and potential stigma associated with adopting a carnivore lifestyle. They offer practical tips for navigating social situations, managing relationships with family and friends who may not understand this way of eating, and finding support within the carnivore community.

**Highlighting Individual Variability and Adaptation:** The sources emphasize that individual responses to a carnivore diet can vary significantly. They discuss factors like genetics, health history, gut microbiome composition, and the importance of a gradual transition to minimize potential side effects.

**Providing Practical Guidance:** The sources offer practical advice for implementing a carnivore diet, including tips on food choices, meal planning, electrolyte management, and addressing potential nutrient deficiencies.

By examining the carnivore diet from various viewpoints and addressing both its potential benefits and challenges, these sources provide a well-rounded perspective that goes beyond simple advocacy. You gain a deeper understanding of the scientific rationale behind this way of eating, the practical considerations for adopting it, and the social and emotional aspects that can influence its success.

# CHAPTER 2

# WHAT & WHY

**Consult with your Physician**

*Note: It's important to consult with a healthcare professional before making any significant dietary changes, especially if you have pre-existing health conditions or are taking medications. The information presented here should not be considered medical advice.*

---

**Contrasting Dietary Approaches: Carnivore vs. Plant-Based**

---

The sources highlight several key differences between the carnivore diet and a plant-based diet, primarily focusing on nutrient profiles, metabolic effects, and potential health outcomes.

## Nutrient Composition and Bioavailability

**Carnivore Diet:** Emphasizes animal-sourced foods like meat, eggs, and seafood, providing a rich source of protein, fat, and certain micronutrients like vitamin B12, heme iron, and zinc. The sources argue that these nutrients are more bioavailable from animal sources, meaning the body can absorb and utilize them more efficiently.

**Plant-Based Diet:** Focuses on plant-derived foods like fruits, vegetables, legumes, grains, and nuts. While rich in fiber, carbohydrates, and various vitamins and minerals, the sources question the bioavailability of certain nutrients like iron and zinc from plant sources, suggesting they may require higher intake to meet the body's needs.

## Macronutrient Ratios and Metabolic Effects

**Carnivore Diet:** Characterized by high protein and fat intake with zero carbohydrates. This macronutrient composition promotes ketosis, a metabolic state where the body shifts from burning glucose to burning fat for fuel. The sources suggest this shift can lead to improved insulin sensitivity, reduced inflammation, and weight loss.

**Plant-Based Diet:** Typically lower in fat and higher in carbohydrates, particularly when including grains and legumes. The sources often express concerns about the potential for high-carbohydrate plant-based diets to contribute to insulin resistance, weight gain, and chronic inflammation.

## Potential Health Outcomes

**Carnivore Diet:** Proponents highlight various potential benefits, including improved metabolic health (reduced blood sugar, improved cholesterol levels, weight loss), reduced inflammation, enhanced mental clarity, and potential reversal of certain chronic conditions like autoimmune diseases and skin issues.

**Plant-Based Diet:** While some individuals may experience health improvements on a plant-based diet, the sources often raise concerns about potential nutrient deficiencies, particularly vitamin B12, iron, and zinc, and suggest that high-carbohydrate plant-based diets could contribute to metabolic dysfunction and chronic disease.

## Digestive Health and the Role of Fiber

**Carnivore Diet:** Eliminates all fiber, which some sources contend is unnecessary and potentially detrimental to gut health. Proponents argue that the human body can thrive without fiber and that eliminating it can improve digestion and reduce bloating.

**Plant-Based Diet:** Emphasizes fiber intake from various plant sources, which is generally considered beneficial for digestive health, promoting regular bowel movements and supporting a healthy gut microbiome.

**Other Notable Differences**

**Social Acceptability and Practicality:** The sources acknowledge that both diets can present social challenges. One source discusses the potential for feeling isolated and judged when adopting a carnivore diet, while other sources mention the difficulties of maintaining a social life that revolves around food. Similarly, individuals following a plant-based diet might also encounter difficulties finding suitable options at social gatherings or restaurants.

**Environmental Impact:** While the sources don't directly compare the environmental impact of the two diets, this is an important consideration. Generally, plant-based diets are considered to have a lower environmental footprint compared to meat-heavy diets.

**Ethical Considerations:** The sources don't extensively discuss ethical considerations related to animal welfare, but this is another important aspect to consider when comparing these two dietary approaches.

## The Nutrient Shift: Why Ex-Vegans Go Carnivore

The sources suggest a compelling reason behind the surprising transition of some ex-vegans to a carnivore diet: the reversal of a nutrient imbalance, particularly concerning the zinc-to-copper ratio.

*Important Note: While the sources offer insights into the experiences of some ex-vegans, it's essential to remember that individual responses to diets can vary greatly. It is crucial to consult with healthcare professionals for personalized dietary guidance.*

**Vegan Diets and Copper Overload:** Vegan diets, rich in grains, legumes, and nuts, tend to be high in copper and low in zinc. This imbalance can be problematic for individuals susceptible to copper accumulation.

**Carnivore Diets as a Counterbalance:** Carnivore diets, with their emphasis on red meat, offer the opposite nutrient profile: high in zinc and low in copper. This shift can help those experiencing copper overload by providing the nutrients needed to regulate copper levels.

**The Impact of Copper Imbalance:** While many individuals tolerate high-copper diets without issues, some are genetically or environmentally predisposed to copper accumulation. Over time, this can lead to various health problems. Switching to a carnivore diet can alleviate these issues by:

The Nutrient Shift: Why Ex-Vegans Go Carnivore Zinc acts as a copper antagonist, helping to balance copper levels in the body.

**Boosting Vitamin A:** Animal-sourced retinol (pre-formed vitamin A) supports ceruloplasmin production, a protein vital for copper metabolism.

This nutritional shift can lead to dramatic improvements in health for those struggling with copper overload, making the carnivore diet appealing despite its stark contrast to veganism.

**Beyond Copper:** The sources also mention the digestive challenges some vegans experience due to the high fiber content of plant-based diets. A carnivore diet, by eliminating fiber, can alleviate these issues for some individuals, leading to improved digestion and reduced bloating.

**The Nutrient Shift:** The sources also observe a trend of carnivores incorporating liver into their diets after a few years. This is attributed to a potential zinc excess and copper deficiency arising from a long-term meat-heavy diet. Liver, being rich in copper, helps to rebalance these levels.

## Reasons for Adopting a Carnivore Diet

*It's important to note that the reasons presented in the sources are largely based on anecdotal evidence, personal experiences, and the perspectives of individuals who advocate for the carnivore diet. While these reasons offer valuable insights into the motivations and beliefs of those who choose this dietary approach, it's crucial to consider these perspectives alongside scientific evidence and guidance from qualified healthcare professionals.*

The sources, primarily featuring proponents of the carnivore diet, offer various reasons why individuals choose this way of eating, often emphasizing its perceived health benefits and its effectiveness in addressing chronic health issues. These reasons can be categorized as follows:

## 1. Healing Chronic Health Conditions:

**Reversing Metabolic Disorders:** The sources strongly advocate for the carnivore diet as a means to address metabolic disorders, including type 2 diabetes, pre-diabetes, and obesity. They argue that the elimination of carbohydrates and the focus on animal-based fats and proteins helps regulate blood sugar levels, improve insulin sensitivity, and promote weight loss.

**Addressing Autoimmune Conditions:** Dr. Ken Berry suggests that many autoimmune conditions improve significantly or even go into remission on a carnivore diet. This is attributed to the diet's anti-inflammatory effects, achieved by eliminating potential dietary triggers like grains, plant oils, and processed foods.

Improving Gut Health: The sources challenge the conventional view that fiber is essential for gut health, arguing that a carnivore diet can actually lead to improved digestion and reduced bloating, gas, and digestive discomfort. They attribute this to the elimination of plant-based fibers, which they suggest can be difficult for humans to digest, and the focus on easily digestible animal proteins and fats.

**2. Weight Loss and Body Composition Changes:**

**Fat Loss and Increased Lean Mass:** The sources consistently highlight the effectiveness of the carnivore diet for weight loss and improving body composition. They attribute this to the diet's ability to reduce insulin levels, promote satiety, and shift the body into a fat-burning state known as ketosis.

**Addressing Specific Body Fat Concerns:** One source, "Hormones guarantee weight loss, calories dont," specifically emphasizes the carnivore diet's ability to target visceral fat, the fat stored around the organs. They argue that by stimulating the hormone glucagon through a high-fat, low-carbohydrate approach, the body becomes more efficient at burning this type of fat.

**3. Mental Clarity, Energy, and Mood Enhancement:**

**Increased Energy Levels:** Individuals often report experiencing increased energy and reduced fatigue after adopting a carnivore diet. The sources attribute this to the sustained energy provided by a diet rich in fat and protein and the elimination of blood sugar fluctuations caused by carbohydrate consumption.

**Improved Mental Clarity and Focus:** The sources suggest that the carnivore diet can enhance mental clarity and focus, attributing these improvements to the stable blood sugar levels, reduced inflammation, and potential benefits for brain health associated with ketosis.

**Mood Stabilization and Reduced Anxiety:** The sources mention that some individuals experience improvements in mood and reduced anxiety on a carnivore diet. While not explicitly stated, this could be linked to the potential benefits of a stable mood and reduced inflammation for mental well-being.

### 4. Simplicity and Dietary Freedom:

**Eliminating Food Choices and Decision Fatigue:** The sources emphasize the simplicity and straightforwardness of the carnivore diet. By limiting food choices to animal products only, individuals eliminate the need for complex meal planning, calorie counting, and navigating a confusing landscape of dietary recommendations.

**Breaking Free from Restrictive Dieting:** The sources suggest that the carnivore diet can be liberating for individuals who have struggled with restrictive diets in the past. They argue that by focusing on satiety and nutrient-dense foods, individuals can break free from the cycle of cravings, deprivation, and guilt often associated with calorie-restricted or low-fat diets.

**5. Alignment with Evolutionary Biology and Human Ancestry**

**The "Proper Human Diet":** The sources, especially Dr. Ken Berry and echoed by the "HomeSteadHow", promote the carnivore diet as the "proper human diet," aligning it with evolutionary biology and the dietary practices of our ancestors. They argue that humans are biologically adapted to thrive on a diet primarily composed of animal products.

## Distinguishing Carnivore from Keto: A Deeper Look

While both carnivore and keto diets share the fundamental principle of minimizing carbohydrate intake to shift the body's metabolism towards fat burning, there are some key distinctions between these two approaches.

### Food Choices and Restrictions

**Carnivore Diet:** As the name suggests, the carnivore diet restricts food choices to animal products only. This means consuming meat (including organ meats), eggs, seafood, and sometimes animal-derived fats like tallow or lard. One source describes the carnivore diet as allowing anything that "runs, creeps, crawls, flies, jumps or swims, or slithers." Plant-based foods, including fruits, vegetables, nuts, seeds, and even dairy products, are strictly excluded.

**Keto Diet:** The ketogenic diet, while also very low in carbohydrates, allows for a wider range of food choices. The emphasis is on consuming high-fat, moderate-protein foods while keeping carbohydrates extremely low (typically under 50 grams per day). One source mentions that keto-friendly foods could include "whole, real, one-ingredient... foods, not keto cookies and cakes and pies and pancakes." This means including non-starchy vegetables, healthy fats (avocados, olive oil, nuts, seeds), and dairy products in addition to meat, eggs, and seafood.

### Stringency and Long-Term Sustainability

**Carnivore Diet:** Known for its extreme restriction, the carnivore diet can be challenging to maintain long-term due to its limited food choices and potential for nutrient deficiencies if not carefully planned. Source 1 highlights some of the "painful lessons" associated with starting a carnivore diet, including the difficulty of eating out and maintaining a social life, potential meat aversion, and the potential for nutrient deficiencies, particularly if organ meats are not included.

**Keto Diet:** The keto diet, while still restrictive, offers more flexibility and variety, making it potentially more sustainable for the long term. However, it requires careful attention to macronutrient ratios and can still pose challenges for individuals accustomed to a standard Western diet high in carbohydrates.

### Impact on Ketosis and Metabolic Adaptation

**Carnivore Diet:** The complete absence of carbohydrates on the carnivore diet ensures a rapid and sustained state of ketosis. The body becomes highly efficient at utilizing fat for fuel, which several sources suggest can have profound benefits for reversing metabolic dysfunction, reducing inflammation, and improving overall health.

**Keto Diet:** The ketogenic diet also induces ketosis, but the process might be slightly slower due to the inclusion of small amounts of carbohydrates from non-starchy vegetables and other permitted foods. The level of ketosis achieved can vary depending on individual carbohydrate tolerance and dietary adherence.

### Potential for Nutrient Deficiencies

**Carnivore Diet:** Due to the exclusion of all plant-based foods, the carnivore diet carries a higher risk of nutrient deficiencies, particularly if not carefully planned to include a variety of animal products, including organ meats. One source points out that some individuals who adopt a carnivore diet might experience zinc excess and copper deficiency, which could be addressed by incorporating liver into the diet.

**Keto Diet:** While a well-formulated ketogenic diet can provide a wide array of nutrients, some individuals might still need to supplement certain vitamins and minerals, depending on their individual needs and food choices.

## Ethical and Environmental Considerations

**Carnivore Diet:** The carnivore diet raises ethical concerns about animal welfare and environmental sustainability, particularly when considering the significant resources required for animal agriculture.

**Keto Diet:** Depending on the specific food choices, a ketogenic diet can have varying impacts on the environment. Including more plant-based fats and proteins can reduce the environmental footprint compared to a more meat-centric approach.

## Choosing the Right Approach

The decision of whether to follow a carnivore or keto diet depends on individual goals, health conditions, preferences, and ethical considerations. It is crucial to thoroughly research both approaches, consult with a qualified healthcare professional, and prioritize nutrient adequacy and long-term sustainability.

# CHAPTER 3

# EVIDENCE

## Benefits of a Carnivore Diet: A Look at the Transformations

The sources provide a wealth of information about the potential benefits people experience after transitioning to a carnivore diet. These benefits span physical, mental, and emotional realms and often interweave, leading to a holistic sense of well-being.

### Physical Transformations

**Weight Loss and Body Composition:** The sources consistently emphasize the effectiveness of the carnivore diet for shedding excess weight and improving body composition. Individuals often report significant reductions in body fat, particularly stubborn visceral fat, and a noticeable increase in lean muscle mass. Dr. Ken Berry suggests that this is linked to the diet's ability to reverse hyperinsulinemia, a condition where insulin levels are chronically elevated, promoting fat storage.

**Reduced Inflammation:** The anti-inflammatory nature of the carnivore diet is a prominent theme throughout the sources. By eliminating inflammatory foods like grains, seed oils, and sugar, the body can reduce chronic inflammation, leading to a cascade of positive effects. Many individuals experience relief from chronic pain, improved joint health, and a reduction in skin issues like eczema and psoriasis.

**Improved Digestion:** While initial adaptation may involve digestive changes like diarrhea or constipation, the sources suggest that long-term carnivore adherence can lead to optimal digestion and bowel function. The absence of plant fiber, often touted for digestive health, allows the body to process food through alternative mechanisms, leading to smooth, regular bowel movements and reduced bloating.

**Enhanced Energy and Sleep:** Many individuals report experiencing a surge in energy and mental clarity after transitioning to a carnivore diet. This is attributed to the body's shift to using ketones, derived from fat, as a more stable and efficient fuel source. Stable blood sugar levels, resulting from eliminating carbohydrate fluctuations, contribute to sustained energy throughout the day without the typical crashes associated with sugar consumption. Additionally, individuals often experience deeper and more restorative sleep, waking up feeling refreshed and revitalized.

**Hormonal Balance:** The sources suggest that the carnivore diet can positively impact hormonal health, particularly for men experiencing low testosterone. The diet's richness in cholesterol, the building block for testosterone, can contribute to increased testosterone levels. Women with PCOS may also benefit from reduced testosterone levels, while others may see slight increases. The diet's impact on insulin sensitivity can also play a role in balancing other hormones, contributing to improved menstrual cycles and reduced symptoms related to hormonal imbalances.

**Increased Nutrient Absorption:** By eliminating plant compounds that can interfere with nutrient absorption, such as phytates and oxalates, the carnivore diet allows for better assimilation of nutrients from animal foods. This can lead to improvements in iron levels, B12 status, and other essential nutrients, addressing deficiencies common in those following restrictive diets.

**Improved Blood Markers:** The sources highlight the potential for the carnivore diet to improve various blood markers associated with health. These include reduced triglycerides, improved cholesterol profiles (increased HDL and decreased LDL), lower fasting insulin levels, and a decrease in inflammatory markers like C-reactive protein (CRP). Dr. Ken Berry encourages individuals to get a comprehensive blood panel before and after starting the diet to track these changes.

**Mental and Emotional Benefits:**

**Enhanced Mental Clarity and Focus:** Many individuals report experiencing a "brain fog lifting" effect after adopting a carnivore diet. The stable blood sugar levels and efficient energy production from ketones contribute to improved cognitive function, allowing for greater focus, concentration, and mental agility.

**Mood Stabilization and Reduced Anxiety:** The sources suggest a link between the carnivore diet and improvements in mood and anxiety levels. This is attributed to the diet's ability to reduce inflammation, balance blood sugar, and potentially influence neurotransmitter production. Individuals often report feeling calmer, more balanced, and less susceptible to mood swings.

**Increased Libido:** Several sources mention a noticeable increase in libido, particularly for men, after transitioning to a carnivore diet. This is likely related to the increase in testosterone levels and overall improvement in hormonal balance.

**Long-Term Lifestyle Changes**

**Reduced Food Cravings and Addictions:** One of the remarkable benefits of the carnivore diet is its potential to break free from food cravings and addictions. By eliminating processed foods, sugar, and refined carbohydrates, the body's dependence on these substances diminishes, leading to a natural decrease in cravings. Individuals often find that they are no longer driven by unhealthy food desires and can make food choices based on nourishment rather than compulsion.

**Shifting Away from Diet Culture:** The sources advocate for a shift away from the restrictive and often harmful mindset of diet culture. By focusing on nutrient-dense foods that satisfy the body's needs, individuals can cultivate a healthier relationship with food, moving beyond the cycle of restriction and binging.

**Mindset Shifts and Personal Growth:** Embracing a carnivore diet often leads to a deeper understanding of the interconnectedness of physical, mental, and emotional well-being. The sources encourage individuals to explore the mindset shifts that can support long-term adherence and overall health. This may involve incorporating practices like meditation, mindfulness, and self-reflection to address any underlying emotional patterns contributing to unhealthy habits.

---

**Insights from "Humans Aren't Omnivores"**

---

The video "Humans Aren't Omnivores" argues against the common belief that humans are biologically designed to consume a mixed diet of plants and animals.

The video ultimately makes a strong case for the carnivore diet, suggesting that aligning our food choices with our evolutionary history may lead to better health outcomes.

Here are three key takeaways:

## Humans are biologically more similar to carnivores than herbivores

The video examines the anatomical and physiological characteristics of the human digestive system, highlighting similarities to carnivores. For example, the video notes that humans lack a cecum, an anatomical feature crucial for herbivores to break down plant fiber. The small intestine length, stomach acidity, and limited jaw motion are also cited as evidence for human carnivory.

## Human evolution points to a meat-centric diet

The video traces human evolution back to Australopithecus, whose tool usage suggests a reliance on hunting and consuming meat. The video argues that our ancestors ate mostly meat and animal products, with minimal plant consumption occurring only between successful hunts. The video also connects the Agricultural Revolution, a period marked by increased plant consumption, with a decrease in human brain size and the emergence of various diseases.

## Modern diets contradict our evolutionary history

The video emphasizes that our modern diets, which are heavily reliant on processed foods and plants, are incompatible with our biological design. This mismatch, the video argues, contributes to various modern health problems. This echoes the themes discussed in our conversation history, where we explored the detrimental effects of high carbohydrate consumption and the benefits of prioritizing fat as a primary fuel source.

---

## Evidence Supporting a Primarily Carnivorous Human Evolutionary History

---

The sources, primarily featuring proponents of the carnivore diet, put forth several arguments to support the claim that humans evolved as primarily carnivorous beings:

### Anatomical and Physiological Features

- **Digestive Tract Similarities to Carnivores:** Source 37 meticulously compares the digestive systems of carnivores and herbivores, highlighting that humans possess several features aligning them more closely with carnivores. These include a highly acidic stomach (pH 1-2), a relatively short small intestine, and the lack of a functional cecum, which is essential for fermenting plant fiber. The source argues that these anatomical characteristics suggest humans are better equipped to digest meat than plant matter.

- **Bicuspid Teeth and Limited Jaw Motion:** Source 44 points out that human teeth are bicuspid, meaning they have ridges that limit side-to-side jaw motion, hindering the efficient grinding of fibrous plant material. This dental structure, the source contends, favors a carnivorous diet focused on tearing and chewing meat.

### Anthropological Evidence

- **Evolutionary Timeline:** Source 46 traces the human lineage back to Miocene hominids, akin to apes and chimps, acknowledging a period of significant fruit and fiber consumption. However, it emphasizes a shift towards meat consumption with the emergence of

32

Australopithecus, who, despite primarily grazing on leaves, began using tools to kill animals. This marks the beginning of a trend towards increased meat consumption throughout human evolution.

- **Early and Middle Pleistocene Homo Sapiens:** Source 47 highlights that during the Ice Age, with the rise of early Homo sapiens like Homo habilis, Homo erectus, and Homo rudolphensis, brain size dramatically increased, coinciding with a greater reliance on tools and hunting. This trend intensified with middle Pleistocene Homo sapiens, including Neanderthals, who engaged in extensive hunting and exhibited a diet primarily composed of meat, evidenced by stable nitrogen isotope studies indicating an 80% meat-based diet.

- **Modern Homo Sapiens:** Source 48 states that early modern Homo sapiens also relied heavily on meat, displaying similar stable nitrogen isotope patterns as Neanderthals. The source suggests that the Agricultural Revolution, while allowing for larger civilizations, marked a turning point where brain size decreased and diseases like tooth decay and gum inflammation emerged, possibly linked to increased plant consumption.

**Historical Accounts and Examples**

- **Ethiopian King's Account:** Source 49 recounts a historical anecdote from Herodotus, describing a conversation between the Ethiopian King and the Persian King. The Ethiopian King, whose people subsisted on boiled meat, blood, and milk, expressed astonishment at the Persian's 70-80 year lifespan, claiming his people lived to 120 or more. While anecdotal, this account is presented as evidence for the potential longevity benefits of a carnivore diet, aligning with genomic data suggesting a human lifespan of 120-150 years.

- **Mongolian Empire:** Source 50 discusses the Mongolian Empire's success as potentially linked to their heavily carnivorous diet, consisting of horse meat and blood. Their dominance and thriving on this diet are presented as further support for the advantages of a meat-based approach.

**Key Points and Counterarguments**

The sources present a compelling case for humans having evolved as primarily carnivorous. However, it's crucial to acknowledge that this perspective is not universally accepted within the scientific community. While the sources provide evidence to support their claims, they primarily represent a pro-carnivore stance and may not fully address alternative interpretations or counterarguments.

It's important to remember that:

- **Dietary Adaptation:** Humans are adaptable and can thrive on a variety of diets. While a carnivore diet might offer benefits for some, it may not be optimal or necessary for everyone.
- **Balanced Perspective:** Considering a range of scientific perspectives and research on human evolution and diet is crucial for forming a comprehensive understanding of this complex topic.

Ultimately, exploring the evidence from various sources and perspectives will enable you to develop a more informed understanding of the role of meat consumption throughout human history and its potential implications for modern-day dietary choices.

## Examples of Carnivorous Diets in History

The sources provide a few notable examples of cultures throughout history that seemingly thrived on predominantly carnivorous diets:

**The Mongols:** The Mongols, renowned for their military prowess and the establishment of the largest contiguous empire in history, stand out as a prime example of a culture that flourished on a heavily meat-based diet. As mentioned in our previous conversation, the Mongols relied heavily on their livestock, particularly horses, for sustenance. Their diet primarily consisted of horse meat, blood, and fermented milk products. Sources 86 and 87 suggest that this carnivorous lifestyle granted them significant logistical advantages in warfare, allowing them to traverse vast distances without being dependent on extensive food supplies. The consumption of horse blood, while seemingly unusual from a modern perspective, likely provided them with readily available nutrients, particularly iron, which could have enhanced their endurance and resilience. One source highlights the Mongols' remarkable success, conquering vast territories across Asia and Europe, suggesting that their meat-centered diet potentially played a crucial role in their military dominance.

**The Ethiopian King's Account:** One source recounts a historical anecdote involving a Persian emissary visiting the king of Ethiopia. The Ethiopian king, upon learning that the Persians primarily consumed bread made from wheat and lived to an average age of 70, expressed amusement, stating, "Well, no wonder you live such short lives if all you eat is dirt." He then contrasted this with his own people's diet, consisting mainly of boiled meat, milk, and blood from their livestock, claiming that they lived to 120 years or more. This account, while potentially embellished, provides a glimpse into a culture that seemingly thrived on a heavily carnivorous diet and attributed their longevity and vitality to their meat-centric lifestyle.

**Native Americans:** Before the introduction of European agricultural practices, many Native American tribes, particularly those inhabiting the Great Plains, subsisted on a diet primarily composed of bison meat. Two sources highlight the practice of driving bison herds over cliffs, providing a substantial source of meat that could sustain these tribes. Another source further elaborates on their impressive physical characteristics, describing them as "tall, strong, and muscular," attributes potentially linked to their high-protein, high-fat diet. The sources also suggest that the adoption of a Western diet, rich in processed foods and refined carbohydrates, led to a significant decline in the health of these populations, with increased rates of obesity, diabetes, and other chronic diseases, further supporting the notion that their traditional meat-based diet was more aligned with their biological needs.

These historical examples, as presented in the sources, suggest that a carnivorous diet was not only feasible but potentially advantageous for certain cultures throughout history. It's crucial to acknowledge, however, that these accounts often highlight specific aspects of these cultures and their dietary practices, potentially overlooking other factors that contributed to their success or longevity.

## Carnivore Diet and Mood: Reported Effects on Well-being

The sources offer various insights into how individuals following a carnivore diet report the impact of this dietary approach on their mood and overall sense of well-being.

### 1. Improved Mental Clarity and Reduced Brain Fog

"HomeSteadHow" highlights that a common experience among carnivore dieters is the dissipation of brain fog, with mental clarity improving significantly around three weeks into the diet. This coincides with the timeframe when the body typically enters ketosis, suggesting a connection between the metabolic shift and enhanced cognitive function.

Aaron Edwards, sharing his experience after six months on a carnivore diet, describes a significant improvement in mental clarity, allowing him to focus and think more effectively.

Richard Smith, reflecting on his transition from a vegan diet to a carnivore approach, expresses a feeling of mental clarity and liberation from the "fog" that he experienced previously.

### 2. Reduced Anxiety and Depression

"HomeSteadHow" notes that many individuals report an improvement in their mood, with a noticeable reduction in anxiety and depression after starting a carnivore diet, often experiencing a "whoa" moment around the three-week mark. This timeframe aligns with the reported improvements in gut health and microbiome balance, suggesting a potential link between these factors and mental well-being.

"HomeSteadHow" also emphasizes the role of the vagus nerve in connecting the gut and the brain, explaining how imbalances in the gut microbiome can negatively impact mental health. By promoting a healthier gut environment, a carnivore diet may help regulate the vagus nerve and improve mood regulation.

"Felix Harder" points out that many ex-vegans, who often struggle with copper overload due to a high intake of plant-based copper sources, experience relief from anxiety and depression after switching to a carnivore diet. This suggests that addressing nutrient imbalances, particularly copper toxicity, can contribute to improved mental well-being.

Shawn Baker, MD, in conversation with "High Intensity Health", observes that studies are increasingly finding a correlation between vegan and vegetarian diets and higher rates of mental health issues, including depression, anxiety, and suicidal ideation. This further supports the notion that eliminating plant-based foods may have positive implications for mental health.

Kent Carnivore attributes the mood-boosting effects of a carnivore diet to the elimination of "anti-nutrients" found in plants, which he believes can disrupt neurotransmitter function and contribute to mood disorders.

### 3. Increased Energy Levels and Vitality

Several sources emphasize the boost in energy levels experienced by individuals on a carnivore diet, attributing this to the body's transition to burning fat for fuel, the elimination of sugar crashes, and improved metabolic efficiency.

"Steak and Butter Gal" describes her experience with increased energy and stamina, allowing her to engage in physical activity more easily and without feeling fatigued.

"HomeSteadHow" highlights the sustained energy levels provided by a carnivore diet, contrasting it with the fluctuating energy patterns often associated with high-carbohydrate diets.

Aaron Edwards reports feeling more energetic and alive after transitioning to a carnivore diet, attributing this to improved nutrient absorption and hormonal balance.

## 4. Reduced Stress and Improved Sleep Quality

While not explicitly addressing stress levels, the sources suggest that the improved mental clarity, reduced anxiety, and increased energy associated with a carnivore diet can indirectly contribute to a greater sense of calm and reduced stress.

"HomeSteadHow" explains that a carnivore diet can help regulate cortisol levels, a key stress hormone, by stabilizing blood sugar and improving insulin sensitivity.

"HomeSteadHow" also discusses the importance of sleep for mental and emotional well-being, suggesting that a carnivore diet can improve sleep quality by reducing inflammation, balancing hormones, and promoting gut health.

Richard Smith shares his experience with reduced anxiety and improved sleep after adopting a carnivore diet, attributing these benefits to the elimination of plant-based foods that he believes were disrupting his sleep patterns.

## 5. Enhanced Sense of Satisfaction and Well-being

Beyond specific mood improvements, the sources highlight a general sense of satisfaction, contentment, and overall well-being reported by carnivore dieters.

"Steak and Butter Gal" describes the profound emotional benefits she has experienced on a carnivore diet, feeling more grounded, balanced, and connected to her body.

Aaron Edwards expresses a sense of deep satisfaction and fulfillment with his carnivore lifestyle, noting that he feels better than he has in years.

"HomeSteadHow" emphasizes the importance of mindset and personal growth within the carnivore journey, suggesting that the dietary changes can create an opportunity for individuals to cultivate greater self-awareness, resilience, and emotional well-being.

It's important to acknowledge that these reported effects on mood and well-being are based on personal experiences and anecdotal evidence. While these accounts provide valuable insights, further research is needed to fully understand the mechanisms underlying these effects and to determine the long-term impact of a carnivore diet on mental health.

# CHAPTER 4

# LIFESTYLE

## Social Challenges on the Carnivore Diet

The sources describe a number of social challenges that individuals often face when they begin a carnivore diet:

**Feeling Isolated and Alone:** The carnivore diet is not mainstream, so individuals may feel like they are the only ones they know who are following this way of eating. They might feel like "an alien in [their] real life as the only carnivore [they] know." It may be challenging to find information and support, especially in the beginning.

Being Judged and Criticized: Individuals often face judgment and criticism from friends, family, and society in general. People who don't understand the diet might question their choices and make comments about their health. They might even criticize a person's character for choosing to eat this way. Source 2 describes how some carnivores worry about being perceived as "crazy" like "those crazy vegans".

Difficulty Navigating Social Gatherings: Because so many social occasions involve food that is off-limits on the carnivore diet, these events can be difficult. Even gatherings at restaurants can be challenging, as the menu might not have suitable options and individuals might feel awkward requesting special preparations.

Facing Pushback from the Medical Community: Many doctors and nutritionists may not be supportive of a carnivore diet and might challenge a person's decision to follow this way of eating. It can be frustrating to receive conflicting advice from healthcare professionals, especially when individuals are experiencing positive results from the diet.

The sources highlight the importance of finding support when following a carnivore diet. Connecting with online or in-person communities can help individuals feel less alone and provide a safe space to discuss their experiences. Having access to resources and information from experienced carnivores and medical professionals who are knowledgeable about the diet can also be helpful.

## Social Support and Community

### Connecting with Like-Minded Individuals

The sources acknowledge that adopting a carnivore diet can be challenging, especially given the potential for social judgment and criticism. They encourage individuals to seek out online and in-person communities where they can connect with others who share their dietary approach and provide support and encouragement.

### Finding Shared Experiences and Success Stories

The sources, particularly "Steak and Butter Gal" and "HomeSteadHow," emphasize the importance of sharing experiences and success stories within the carnivore community. These testimonials can inspire and motivate others, especially those new to the diet, by demonstrating the potential benefits and providing a sense of belonging and validation.

**Potential Benefits of a Carnivore Diet for Autoimmune Conditions**

While the sources don't directly focus on specific autoimmune conditions, they offer a general framework for understanding how a carnivore diet might potentially benefit individuals with such conditions. The key concept revolves around the idea that eliminating potential triggers and reducing inflammation are crucial steps in managing autoimmune disorders.

## 1. Eliminating Dietary Triggers

**Plant Compounds as Potential Triggers:** The sources strongly advocate that certain compounds found in plant foods, often referred to as "anti-nutrients" or "toxins," can trigger or exacerbate autoimmune responses in susceptible individuals.

**Examples of Anti-Nutrients:** These compounds include lectins, oxalates, phytates, and tannins. The sources suggest that these substances can disrupt gut health, interfere with nutrient absorption, and stimulate the immune system, potentially contributing to autoimmune flare-ups.

**Individual Sensitivities:** It's important to note that not everyone reacts negatively to these plant compounds. However, the sources suggest that for individuals with autoimmune conditions, eliminating these potential triggers through a carnivore diet could be beneficial.

## 2. Reducing Inflammation

**Chronic Inflammation and Autoimmunity:** Chronic inflammation is a hallmark of autoimmune disorders. The sources posit that a carnivore diet, by eliminating potential inflammatory triggers from plant foods, can help reduce overall inflammation in the body, potentially leading to symptom improvement.

**Insulin and Inflammation:** The sources also link high insulin levels to inflammation. They argue that a carnivore diet, by stabilizing blood sugar and reducing insulin spikes, can further contribute to lowering inflammation.

## 3. Nutrient Density and Gut Health

**Nutrient-Rich Animal Foods:** The sources emphasize the nutrient density of animal foods, particularly meat, organs, and bone marrow. They argue that these foods provide a rich source of essential nutrients, including vitamins, minerals, and amino acids, which are crucial for supporting immune function and overall health.

**Gut Health and Autoimmunity:** The sources acknowledge the importance of gut health in managing autoimmune conditions. While they don't explicitly discuss the impact of a carnivore diet on the gut microbiome, they suggest that eliminating plant fibers and potential irritants could contribute to a healthier gut environment.

**Specific Mentions in the Sources**

**Autoimmune Conditions and Carnivore Diet:** One source explicitly states that people with autoimmune conditions "that they consider

46

chronic and progressive" might experience significant improvement or even remission on a carnivore diet.

**Skin Conditions:** Skin conditions like eczema and psoriasis, often linked to autoimmune dysfunction, tend to improve on a carnivore diet. This improvement is attributed to the elimination of inflammatory triggers and the reduction of chronic inflammation.

**Lymphatic Disorders:** One source presents the experience of a doctor who specializes in lymphatic disorders. She observed "spectacular" improvements in her patients' swelling conditions, even in those without weight loss, when they adopted a ketogenic or carnivore diet. This observation suggests a potential link between these diets and improved lymphatic function.

**Important Considerations**

While the sources offer intriguing insights into the potential benefits of a carnivore diet for managing autoimmune conditions, it's crucial to approach this information with caution:

## Obtaining Vitamin C and Micronutrients from Animal Sources

The sources present a diverse range of viewpoints on the feasibility of acquiring sufficient vitamin C and micronutrients solely from animal food sources.

### Arguments in Favor of Animal Sources Providing Adequate Nutrients

**"Virtually Every Nutrient":** One source boldly claims that properly raised and fed animals, particularly fatty red meat, contain "virtually every nutrient" necessary for human health. This statement encompasses all amino acids, fatty acids, and a significant portion of vitamins and minerals, provided the animals grazed on nutrient-rich soil. This perspective aligns with the argument that humans, as natural carnivores, can derive all their essential nutrients from animal sources.

**Micronutrient-Rich Organ Meats:** Another source highlights the importance of organ meats, especially liver, in a carnivore diet. It suggests that the recent surge in popularity of liver among carnivore enthusiasts could be attributed to a need to address potential copper deficiencies that may arise from a prolonged diet primarily focused on muscle meat. Liver is known to be a rich source of copper, along with other essential vitamins and minerals, further supporting the notion that a diverse range of animal products can provide a comprehensive nutrient profile.

**"Nutrient-Dense Superfood":** Yet another source enthusiastically advocates for red meat as a "nutrient-dense, ancestrally appropriate superfood," particularly when sourced from animals raised on properly treated soil and fed appropriately. This perspective emphasizes the nutritional completeness of meat, suggesting it can fulfill all the body's micronutrient requirements.

### Acknowledging the Vitamin C Debate

**Vitamin C in Meat:** One source acknowledges the common belief that vitamin C is primarily obtained from plants. However, it counters this by stating that vitamin C is also present in animal products, albeit in lower quantities. For example, a 12-ounce beef steak contains approximately 12 milligrams of vitamin C. The source further argues that a low-carbohydrate diet reduces the body's requirement for vitamin C, suggesting that the amount found in meat could be sufficient.

**Potential Nutrient Deficiencies:** Another source presents a more nuanced perspective, acknowledging that while animal sources can provide a wide array of nutrients, individual needs may vary. The source suggests paying attention to cravings, as they could indicate specific nutrient deficiencies. While advocating for prioritizing animal-based foods, it suggests incorporating plant-based foods if a strong craving persists to address potential nutrient gaps.

### Addressing Potential Concerns

Soil Quality and Nutrient Content: Several sources emphasize the importance of consuming animals raised on nutrient-rich soil. The concern is that modern agricultural practices often deplete soil quality, potentially impacting the nutrient content of meat. This highlights the need for responsible farming practices and conscious sourcing of animal products to ensure optimal nutrient intake.

**Balancing Zinc and Copper:** One source cautions against potential copper deficiencies that may arise from a long-term carnivore diet heavily focused on muscle meat. It suggests that the high zinc content in muscle meat can, over time, lead to an imbalance in the zinc-to-copper ratio. Incorporating copper-rich organ meats, like liver, can help mitigate this potential issue.

**Bioavailability of Nutrients:** While some sources assert that meat offers superior bioavailability of certain nutrients compared to plant sources, the broader scientific community recognizes that bioavailability can vary depending on the specific nutrient, food source, and individual factors.

**Summary**

The sources present a compelling case for the potential of obtaining sufficient vitamin C and micronutrients from animal sources. However, they also highlight certain caveats, emphasizing the importance of consuming animals raised on nutrient-rich soil, incorporating organ meats for a balanced nutrient profile, and paying attention to individual needs and potential deficiencies. The broader scientific community continues to debate the optimal human diet, with varying perspectives on the role and sufficiency of animal-based foods in meeting all nutrient requirements.

## Common Arguments Against the Carnivore Diet and Their Counterarguments

The sources address several common criticisms leveled against the carnivore diet, offering insights into how proponents of this way of eating respond to these concerns.

**Social Isolation and Judgment:** The carnivore diet, being a significant departure from mainstream dietary norms, can lead to feelings of isolation and social judgment. Source 1 acknowledges this challenge, noting that starting a carnivore diet can feel like "stepping into a whole new world," especially when facing a lack of understanding and support from friends and family. The source suggests that recognizing and preparing for potential social awkwardness and criticism can help individuals navigate these situations. Source 1 also highlights the importance of finding online or in-person carnivore communities for support and connection, suggesting that sharing experiences and learning from others who have successfully adopted this lifestyle can mitigate feelings of loneliness.

**Difficulty with Social Outings and Restaurant Dining:** The restrictive nature of the carnivore diet can pose challenges when participating in social gatherings or dining out. Source 2 acknowledges this, stating that many social events revolve around foods incompatible with a carnivore diet. However, the source offers practical solutions, such as bringing carnivore-friendly foods to gatherings or calling restaurants in advance to inquire about plain meat preparation options. The source emphasizes that maintaining a social life while adhering to a carnivore diet is possible with some planning and communication.

51

**Nutrient Deficiencies (Especially Fiber and Vitamin C)**

Perhaps the most common criticism of the carnivore diet centers around potential nutrient deficiencies, particularly concerning fiber and vitamin C, which are generally absent in animal-based foods.

**Fiber:** Multiple sources challenge the widely held belief that fiber is essential for human health, particularly for digestion. They argue that the human body can function effectively without fiber and suggest that excessive fiber consumption might even be detrimental to gut health. Source 48 cites personal experiences with improved digestion and reduced gastrointestinal issues after eliminating fiber from their diet, suggesting that fiber might not be as crucial as conventionally believed. Source 9 further supports this perspective, stating that medical professionals often perpetuate misinformation about the necessity of fiber due to inadequate training in nutrition.

**Vitamin C:** One source directly addresses the concern regarding vitamin C deficiency on a carnivore diet. It counters the prevalent notion that vitamin C is exclusively found in plants, claiming that animal products also contain vitamin C, albeit in smaller amounts. The source suggests that a low-carbohydrate diet, like the carnivore diet, reduces the body's requirement for vitamin C, implying that the amount found in meat could be sufficient. Another source further challenges the emphasis on plant sources for vitamin C, pointing to the historical rise in macular degeneration, a condition often linked to vitamin C deficiency, coinciding with the introduction of processed foods and seed oils. It implies that these dietary changes, rather than a lack of plant consumption, might be contributing to such deficiencies.

**Negative Health Impacts (Cholesterol, Heart Disease, Kidney Problems)**

Concerns about the potential negative health impacts of a carnivore diet, particularly regarding cholesterol levels, heart disease, and kidney function, are often raised.

**Cholesterol and Heart Health:** Two sources counter the fear surrounding saturated fat and cholesterol commonly associated with meat consumption. Another source delves into the scientific evidence challenging the link between saturated fat and cholesterol, arguing that this connection has been largely debunked. Yet another source suggests that the demonization of saturated fat and cholesterol stems from a misunderstanding of how these substances function in the body. It emphasizes the importance of differentiating between dietary cholesterol and cholesterol produced by the body, suggesting that dietary cholesterol has minimal impact on blood cholesterol levels. Source 82 further reinforces this perspective, arguing that the root cause of heart disease lies in inflammation and insulin resistance often triggered by processed foods and excessive sugar consumption, not cholesterol from animal products.

**Kidney Health:** The argument that a high-protein diet, like the carnivore diet, can harm kidney function is directly addressed in one source. This source presents personal experience as evidence, stating that their kidney function, as measured by creatinine and eGFR levels, actually improved after adopting a carnivore diet. This example challenges the notion that high protein intake necessarily leads to kidney damage, suggesting that a meat-based diet might not be detrimental to kidney health, as commonly perceived.

**Ethical and Environmental Concerns**

Beyond potential health implications, critics often raise ethical and environmental concerns regarding a carnivore diet.

**Animal Welfare:** The ethical implications of consuming animal products are a significant point of contention, particularly for individuals concerned about animal welfare. The sources, however, generally adopt a pragmatic approach, acknowledging the reality of the food chain and emphasizing the importance of responsible and humane animal husbandry practices. Source 70 highlights the role of grazing animals in maintaining healthy ecosystems, suggesting that raising livestock for meat consumption can be compatible with environmental sustainability.

**Environmental Impact:** The environmental impact of animal agriculture is another major criticism leveled against the carnivore diet. Critics argue that raising livestock for meat production contributes significantly to greenhouse gas emissions, deforestation, and resource depletion. The sources, however, offer counterarguments, highlighting the potential for regenerative grazing practices to mitigate environmental damage and even contribute to carbon sequestration. Source 92 emphasizes the need to shift the focus from simply reducing meat consumption to promoting sustainable and regenerative farming practices, suggesting that responsible animal agriculture can be part of a solution to environmental challenges.

# CHAPTER 5

# ADOPTING

## Important Considerations

**Individual Variability:** It's crucial to remember that everyone responds differently to dietary changes. The benefits experienced on a carnivore diet can vary significantly depending on individual factors, including previous diet and lifestyle, metabolic health, underlying conditions, and adherence to the diet.

**Consultation with Healthcare Professionals:** Seeking guidance from healthcare professionals knowledgeable about low-carbohydrate and carnivore diets is essential, especially for individuals with pre-existing health conditions or taking medications.

**Potential for Nutrient Deficiencies:** While the carnivore diet is rich in many nutrients, there is a potential for deficiencies in certain vitamins and minerals, particularly if organ meats are not included. Regular monitoring of nutrient levels and supplementation, if necessary, is important.

---

**Adapting to a Carnivore Diet: A Timeline**

---

The sources offer varying perspectives on the adaptation period for a carnivore diet, highlighting both short-term adjustments and long-term transformations. While some benefits are experienced quickly, fully reaping the rewards can be a gradual process.

### Initial Adaptation (2-6 Weeks)

The initial phase of adapting to a carnivore diet can present challenges as the body adjusts to the absence of carbohydrates and a significant increase in fat intake. This period often involves:

- **Digestive Changes:** Fluctuations in bowel movements, including constipation or diarrhea, are common as the digestive system acclimates to the lack of fiber and increased fat.

- **Electrolyte Imbalances:** A shift in fluid balance due to reduced insulin levels can lead to the excretion of excess water and electrolytes, potentially resulting in symptoms like muscle cramps, headaches, and fatigue. This phase is often referred to as the "keto flu".

- **Carbohydrate Cravings:** Intense cravings for sugar and processed foods can arise as the body withdraws from its dependence on carbohydrates.

**Homeostasis and Initial Benefits (3 Weeks - Several Months)**

As the body becomes accustomed to burning fat for fuel (keto-adaptation), individuals often start experiencing the positive effects of the carnivore diet. These benefits include:

- **Reduced Inflammation:** The sources consistently highlight the anti-inflammatory effects of the carnivore diet, which can lead to the alleviation of chronic pain, improved skin health, and a general sense of well-being.

- **Increased Energy and Mental Clarity:** Many individuals report experiencing a surge in energy, improved focus, and reduced brain fog as their bodies adapt to using ketones for fuel.

- **Mood Improvement:** Some individuals observe a stabilization of mood and a reduction in anxiety, potentially linked to the diet's impact on inflammation, blood sugar regulation, and neurotransmitter production.

- **Weight Loss and Body Composition Changes:** The sources emphasize the carnivore diet's effectiveness for fat loss and improved body composition, often citing significant reductions in body fat and increases in lean muscle mass.

**Continued Healing and Optimization (6 Months - 2 Years)**

The sources suggest that the benefits of the carnivore diet continue to unfold over time as the body undergoes cellular renewal and deeper healing. This extended period may involve:

- **Cellular Turnover and Mitochondrial Biogenesis:** The body gradually replaces damaged cells with healthier ones, and the number and efficiency of mitochondria (the energy powerhouses of cells) increase.

- **Further Reduction in Autoimmune Markers:** Individuals with autoimmune conditions may observe continued improvement in their symptoms and a reduction in inflammatory markers.

- **Stabilization of Digestion and Bowel Function:** As the gut microbiome adjusts to the absence of plant fibers, bowel movements become more regular and digestive discomfort diminishes.

**Long-Term Maintenance and Mindset Shifts (Beyond 2 Years)**

The sources emphasize that adopting a carnivore diet is not simply a short-term fix but a lifestyle change that requires ongoing commitment and mindset shifts.

- **Reduced Food Cravings and Increased Satiety:** Individuals often find that their cravings for processed foods and sugar diminish over time as their bodies become accustomed to a nutrient-dense, satiating diet.

- **Shifting Away from Diet Culture:** The sources encourage a move away from restrictive dieting and a focus on nourishing the body with foods that promote health and well-being.

- **Addressing Underlying Mental and Emotional Patterns:** The sources acknowledge that dietary changes can be intertwined with mental and emotional well-being, encouraging individuals to address any underlying patterns that may contribute to unhealthy eating habits.

**Individual Variability**

It's crucial to recognize that the adaptation timeline for a carnivore diet can vary significantly depending on individual factors, including:

- **Previous Diet and Lifestyle:** Individuals transitioning from a highly processed, high-carbohydrate diet may experience more pronounced withdrawal symptoms and a longer adaptation period compared to those already following a low-carbohydrate or ketogenic diet.

- **Metabolic Health and Underlying Conditions:** Individuals with metabolic disorders or chronic health conditions may experience faster or slower healing depending on the severity of their condition and their individual responses to the diet.

- **Adherence to the Diet:** Strict adherence to a carnivore diet, eliminating all plant-based foods, is often emphasized for optimal adaptation and results.

## Negative Symptoms When Starting a Carnivore Diet

The sources detail a variety of unpleasant symptoms that individuals may experience, especially in the initial stages of the carnivore diet.

While these sources highlight potential negative experiences, they generally present them as temporary and surmountable hurdles on the path to the perceived long-term benefits of a carnivore diet.

**Digestive Issues**

**Diarrhea:** The sudden shift to a high-fat, zero-fiber diet can disrupt bowel movements, leading to diarrhea in some individuals. One source suggests that this may occur when individuals consume more fat than their bodies can handle at the moment and advises temporarily reducing fat intake or opting for cold or room-temperature fats to help alleviate symptoms. Another source links diarrhea on the carnivore diet to an electrolyte imbalance and encourages increasing salt intake to resolve the issue. Yet another source, drawing on personal experience, notes that diarrhea is common in the beginning stages but eventually resolves as the body adapts to digesting primarily fat.

**Constipation:** Conversely, some individuals might experience constipation. One source recommends increasing salt or fat consumption to stimulate digestion and alleviate constipation.

**Bloating:** While one source claims that bloating goes away completely on the carnivore diet due to the body adjusting to digesting primarily one type of food, another source notes this as a possible initial symptom, suggesting that there may be an adjustment period for the digestive system.

## Oxalate Dumping

**Joint and Muscle Aches:** As the body adjusts to eliminating oxalates, individuals may experience aches in their joints and muscles. This is a detoxification process as the body purges stored oxalates, which are compounds found in many plant foods.

**Skin Issues:** Worsening of existing skin problems or development of new rashes is also possible during oxalate dumping. The source notes that skin issues might get worse before they get better as the body detoxifies.

**Cloudy Urine:** Cloudy urine can be a symptom of oxalate dumping, indicating the body is working to flush out these crystals.

## "Keto Flu" or Carb Withdrawal

**Lower Energy and Fatigue:** Individuals may feel tired and drained as their bodies transition from burning glucose to burning fat for fuel.

**Muscle Cramps:** Electrolyte imbalances during this transition can cause muscle cramping.

**Headaches:** Similar to muscle cramps, headaches during the initial phase of the carnivore diet may be linked to electrolyte depletion as the body adapts to a low-carb state.

## Mental and Emotional Challenges

**Food Cravings:** Intense cravings for sugar, processed foods, and other comfort foods are a common challenge, particularly in the beginning. One source suggests that these intense cravings can be attributed to carbohydrate addiction and that the body will experience withdrawal symptoms as it adjusts to a lack of carbs.

**Meat Aversion:** Some individuals develop an aversion to meat, possibly stemming from the monotony of consuming it frequently.

**Feeling Alone and Judged:** As mentioned earlier, these social challenges can have an impact on mental and emotional well-being. Feeling isolated or judged for dietary choices can lead to stress, anxiety, and frustration.

It's important to remember that these symptoms are typically temporary and tend to subside as the body adapts to the carnivore diet. Sources offer various strategies for managing these challenges, including:

- **Electrolyte Supplementation:** Increasing salt intake and considering electrolyte supplements can help mitigate symptoms like muscle cramps, headaches, and fatigue.
- **Managing Oxalate Dumping:** Gradually transitioning to a carnivore diet, rather than making a sudden switch, may help minimize the severity of oxalate dumping symptoms.
- **Finding Support:** Joining online or in-person communities can provide emotional support and practical advice for dealing with cravings and navigating social situations.

## Two Approaches to Oxalate Dumping

Source explains that oxalate dumping occurs when individuals transition to a carnivore diet after consuming a diet high in oxalates. Oxalates are tiny crystals that accumulate in the body and can cause a range of symptoms like:

- Aches in joints and muscles.
- Rashes and worsening of skin issues before they get better.
- Cloudy urine.

Foods that are high in oxalates, include:

- Sweet potatoes
- Spices like black pepper and cinnamon
- Certain leafy greens like kale and spinach
- Nuts and grains

The source notes that when someone stops consuming these high-oxalate foods, the body attempts to eliminate the stored oxalates, resulting in the unpleasant symptoms associated with oxalate dumping.

One Source presents two contrasting approaches to managing oxalate dumping:

**Gradual Transition:** This approach involves slowly weaning off oxalate-heavy foods and gradually easing into a full carnivore lifestyle. By doing so, individuals can lessen the severity of oxalate dumping symptoms that often affect those who abruptly adopt a carnivore diet.

**Using "Crutches":** This approach involves temporarily consuming small amounts of high-oxalate foods to mitigate the harsh symptoms of oxalate dumping. These "crutches" essentially help the body adjust to the lower oxalate intake more gradually. Examples include:

• Lemon juice as a dipping sauce for meat.

• Coffee.

• Black pepper.

• Chocolate (cautioned against due to potential for overconsumption).

This source ultimately recommends the slow transition as the most effective approach to overcoming oxalate dumping.

## Managing Cravings on the Carnivore Diet

The sources highlight the significance of cravings when transitioning to a carnivore diet and offer various strategies for managing them.

The sources demonstrate that successfully navigating the carnivore transition involves recognizing cravings as a natural part of the process. Whether adopting a gradual approach, focusing on electrolyte balance, or understanding potential nutrient deficiencies, the key lies in adopting strategies that support both physical and psychological adaptation.

**Cravings as a Major Challenge:** Several sources emphasize the intensity of cravings, particularly for those accustomed to a standard American diet. These cravings primarily stem from the withdrawal of carbohydrates and sugars, substances to which many individuals develop an addiction. The sources compare these cravings to withdrawal symptoms experienced when quitting nicotine or alcohol.

**Understanding the "Why":** A common strategy for managing cravings involves constantly reminding oneself of the reasons for adopting the carnivore diet. This involves identifying the personal "why," which could be related to healing chronic health issues, achieving specific fitness goals, or simply experiencing improved overall well-being. The stronger the emotional connection to this "why," the more likely it is to help someone overcome cravings.

Here are some contrasting strategies for managing cravings, as presented in the sources:

**Eliminating Temptation:** The most straightforward approach involves removing all tempting foods from the house. This prevents impulsive decisions driven by cravings, especially during moments of stress or exhaustion.

**Designated Fatty Foods:** Another strategy focuses on consuming specific fatty foods when cravings strike. The idea is that fat satiates and helps suppress cravings, particularly for sugar. This could range from eating pure animal fat, like a stick of butter, to consuming boiled eggs topped with butter. The key is to have these foods readily available and cooked, making them easily accessible when cravings hit.

**Gradual Transition:** Some sources suggest a more gradual transition to the carnivore diet to mitigate the intensity of cravings and withdrawal symptoms. This involves slowly weaning off carbohydrate-heavy and oxalate-rich foods, easing the body into the new dietary regime.

**Electrolyte Management:** Ensuring adequate electrolyte intake, particularly sodium, is crucial during the initial adaptation phase. This can help alleviate symptoms associated with carbohydrate withdrawal, including cravings. Consuming high-quality salt, like Redmond Real Salt or Himalayan salt, and considering electrolyte supplements are recommended.

Beyond these strategies, understanding the underlying mechanisms behind cravings is crucial. The sources suggest that:

**Microbiome Influence:** The composition of the gut microbiome can significantly influence cravings. It's theorized that certain microbes thrive on specific foods and can manipulate cravings to ensure their survival. The shift to a carnivore diet, with its reduced carbohydrate intake, can disrupt this balance and lead to intense cravings during the initial adjustment period.

**Nutrient Deficiencies:** While some cravings might indicate an addiction to sugar and carbohydrates, others could signal nutrient deficiencies. This is particularly relevant for ex-vegans transitioning to a carnivore diet. Their previous diet, often rich in copper and low in zinc, can lead to imbalances. A carnivore diet, high in zinc and low in copper, can initially correct this imbalance. However, over time, a strict carnivore diet might lead to a zinc excess and copper deficiency, prompting cravings for foods rich in copper, like liver.

## Rising Glucose and A1c on a Carnivore Diet

The sources and the conversation history do not contain a specific explanation from carnivore diet proponents regarding the observed rise in blood glucose and A1c levels in some individuals following this diet. However, there is information in the sources that may offer some insights into this phenomenon.

It's important to note that these are potential explanations derived from information within the sources. Further research is needed to specifically address the reasons for elevated blood glucose and A1c levels in some individuals following a carnivore diet.

**Adaptive Glucose Sparing:** One source explains a concept known as "adaptive glucose sparing" which occurs when someone has followed a low-carb diet for an extended period and their body has become fat-adapted. In this state, most of the body's cells have adapted to primarily utilize fatty acids and ketones for fuel. This adaptation can sometimes lead to a slight elevation in fasting blood sugar levels, even reaching the upper limits of what is considered normal or the lower end of pre-diabetes.

**Individual Variability in Metabolism:** Another source emphasizes that individual metabolisms vary. While a low-carb diet can improve insulin resistance and diabetes markers for many people, a select percentage do not experience these benefits. The source suggests that the traditional metrics for evaluating blood glucose and A1c levels may not accurately apply to individuals who have adapted to a low-carb or carnivore lifestyle.

**Stress Response and Gluconeogenesis:** In our conversation history, we discussed how the body can produce glucose from protein through a process called gluconeogenesis, particularly during times of stress. One source further elaborates on this, explaining that when carbohydrate intake is very low, the body may increase gluconeogenesis from muscle tissue to meet its glucose needs. This process is driven by hormones like adrenaline and cortisol and can lead to elevated blood sugar levels.

**Impact of Other Factors:** Yet another source highlights the importance of considering various factors that can influence blood glucose levels beyond just dietary carbohydrate intake. These factors include stress, sleep, the timing of food intake, and the presence of other health conditions.

**Potential Need for Re-evaluation of Metrics:** Sever sources suggest that the standard reference ranges for blood glucose and A1c might need to be re-evaluated for individuals on a carnivore or long-term low-carb diet. The current metrics are based on populations consuming a standard Western diet that includes carbohydrates. As individuals adapt to using fat as their primary fuel source, these traditional markers may no longer accurately reflect their metabolic health.

## Adapting to a Carnivore Diet:
## Physiological Shifts and Common Symptoms

The sources offer insights into the body's adaptation process when transitioning to a carnivore diet, highlighting both the physiological changes and the common symptoms experienced during this period.

**Metabolic Shift: From Sugar Burner to Fat Burner**

One of the most significant adaptations involves the body's primary energy source. The sources emphasize that a carnivore diet, devoid of carbohydrates, forces the body to switch from burning glucose (sugar) to burning fat for fuel. This metabolic transition is often referred to as becoming "fat-adapted" or "keto-adapted."

**Ketogenesis and Ketones:** When carbohydrate intake is drastically reduced, the liver begins producing ketones from stored fat. Ketones serve as an alternative energy source for the brain and other organs, effectively replacing glucose.

**Timeline for Adaptation:** While "fat adaptation" occurs relatively quickly, achieving full "keto-adaptation," where the body efficiently utilizes ketones, typically takes longer. The sources suggest an average timeframe of 3-6 months, although individual experiences can vary.

**Enhancing Keto-Adaptation:** One source suggests that high-intensity workouts, such as sprinting or rowing, can accelerate keto-adaptation by increasing the production of monocarboxylate transporters (MCTs). These transporters facilitate the movement of ketones from the liver to target cells, enhancing their utilization.

**Digestive System Adjustments**

Transitioning to a purely animal-based diet also entails significant adjustments for the digestive system:

**Reduced Fiber Intake:** A carnivore diet eliminates fiber, a component humans cannot digest. The sources argue that this lack of fiber leads to several positive changes, including:

- **Improved Digestion and Reduced Bloating:** Several sources report experiencing improved digestion, reduced bloating, and less gas production after adopting a carnivore diet. They attribute this to the absence of fiber, suggesting that humans are better suited to digesting meat than plant matter.

- **Changes in Bowel Movements:** While the sources acknowledge initial fluctuations in bowel movements, such as diarrhea or constipation, they assert that these are temporary adjustments as the digestive system adapts to a high-fat, low-fiber diet. One source suggests that ensuring adequate electrolyte intake can help mitigate these issues.

**Increased Fat Consumption:** The high-fat content of a carnivore diet requires the body to adapt to digesting and utilizing larger amounts of fat. Another source notes that this can initially lead to diarrhea as the body adjusts to processing the increased fat intake.

**The "Carnivore Flu" and Other Adaptation Symptoms**

The adaptation period often involves a range of uncomfortable symptoms collectively known as the "keto flu" or "carnivore flu." These symptoms typically arise as the body transitions from burning glucose to burning fat and can include:

**Lower Energy and Fatigue:** The initial shift away from readily available glucose can lead to feelings of low energy and fatigue. Source 7 suggests embracing rest and sleep during this phase to allow the body to adjust.

**Muscle Cramps:** Electrolyte imbalances, particularly a loss of sodium, potassium, and magnesium, can contribute to muscle cramps. The sources recommend increasing salt intake and supplementing with electrolytes to alleviate this symptom.

**Headaches:** Dehydration and electrolyte imbalances can also trigger headaches during the adaptation phase. Again, staying hydrated and ensuring adequate electrolyte intake are crucial.

**Meat Aversion:** Some individuals might experience a temporary aversion to meat as they adjust to a predominantly meat-based diet. Source 6 suggests combating this by experimenting with different types of meat, cooking methods, and temperatures.

**Oxalate Dumping:** If transitioning from a diet high in oxalates (found in certain plant foods), individuals might experience symptoms like joint pain, rashes, and cloudy urine as the body eliminates stored oxalates. One source suggests a gradual transition to minimize these effects.

**Emotional and Mental Shifts**

Beyond physiological adaptations, the sources also highlight potential emotional and mental changes during the transition:

**Cravings and Withdrawal Symptoms:** Cravings for sugar, junk food, and other comfort foods can be intense, particularly during stressful periods. These cravings are attributed to carbohydrate addiction and withdrawal. The source recommends removing temptations from the environment, focusing on the reasons for adopting the diet, and identifying alternative fatty foods to satisfy cravings.

**Social Challenges:** Multiple sources acknowledge the social difficulties that can arise when adopting a carnivore diet. Feeling isolated, judged, and finding it challenging to participate in social gatherings centered around food are common concerns. The sources recommend connecting with online or local carnivore communities for support and sharing experiences.

**Importance of Patience and Support**

The sources consistently emphasize that the adaptation period is temporary and that symptoms will eventually subside as the body fully transitions to a fat-burning state. Patience, persistence, and seeking support from others who have successfully adopted the diet are key to navigating this phase.

| **Common Blood Work Changes on a Carnivore Diet** |
| --- |

The sources, primarily featuring Dr. Ken Berry, detail several blood work changes commonly observed in individuals following a carnivore diet.

### Complete Blood Count (CBC)

**Improved Anemia:** Dr. Berry notes that many people suffer from anemia due to iron, B12, or folate deficiency. A carnivore diet, rich in these nutrients, often leads to dramatic improvements in anemia markers, specifically hematocrit and hemoglobin, within a few months.

### Complete Metabolic Panel (CMP)

**Improved Liver Function:** For those with fatty liver disease, a carnivore diet can help normalize liver enzymes, specifically AST and ALT, although complete normalization may take longer than three months.

**Improved Kidney Function:** Individuals with chronic kidney disease may see improvements in their creatinine levels and estimated glomerular filtration rate (eGFR) on a carnivore diet, suggesting potential benefits for kidney health.

**Lower Blood Sugar:** The CMP also reveals lower blood sugar levels in individuals who previously had elevated levels, highlighting the diet's effectiveness in regulating blood sugar.

### Urinalysis (UA)

**Presence of Ketones:** Dr. Berry explains that the presence of ketones in the urine is a normal finding on a carnivore diet as it promotes ketosis, a metabolic state where the body burns fat for fuel.

**Lipid Panel**

**Lower Triglycerides:** A carnivore diet, being very low in carbohydrates, typically leads to a decrease in triglycerides, especially if they were elevated before starting the diet.

**Increased HDL Cholesterol:** The "good" cholesterol, HDL, often increases on a carnivore diet if levels were previously low.

**Variable Total and LDL Cholesterol:** Dr. Berry acknowledges that there is variability in how total cholesterol and LDL cholesterol respond to a carnivore diet. About one-third of people experience a decrease, one-third see no change, and one-third have an increase. In a small percentage (1%), these levels can rise significantly, potentially raising concerns for some doctors .

Hemoglobin A1c (HbA1c)

**Lower HbA1c:** This marker, indicating long-term blood sugar control, typically decreases on a carnivore diet, particularly in individuals with pre-diabetes, type 2 diabetes, or type 1 diabetes. Dr. Berry notes that many long-term carnivores achieve HbA1c levels in the healthy range (4.8-5.2).

**Fasting Insulin**

**Reduced Fasting Insulin:** While many doctors don't routinely check this marker, Dr. Berry strongly recommends it. He observes that a carnivore diet typically leads to a significant reduction in fasting insulin levels, which can help protect against numerous chronic diseases .

## Hormone Levels

**Increased Testosterone (Men):** Dr. Berry reports that men often experience an increase in total testosterone levels, ranging from 50 to 350 points, after three months on a carnivore diet.

**Slight Increase in Testosterone (Women):** Women without PCOS may see a slight increase in testosterone. However, women with PCOS tend to experience a decrease in their abnormally high testosterone levels.

**Changes in DHEA:** Similar to testosterone, DHEA levels may increase slightly in healthy individuals but decrease in women with PCOS who typically have elevated levels.

## Inflammatory Markers

**Decreased C-Reactive Protein (CRP):** CRP, a marker of inflammation, typically decreases after three months on a carnivore diet, particularly if it was elevated previously.

## Thyroid Panel

**Normalization of TSH:** Individuals with hypothyroidism may notice a decrease in TSH levels, moving them closer to the normal range.

**Increase in Free T3 and Free T4:** These thyroid hormones may increase in individuals with hypothyroidism, potentially allowing them to reduce their thyroid medication dosage.

**Decreased Thyroid Antibodies:** People with Hashimoto's thyroiditis, characterized by elevated thyroid antibodies (TPO and TG), often see a reduction in these antibodies after three months on a carnivore diet

## Blood pH

**Stable Blood pH:** Contrary to the common myth that eating meat makes the body acidic, Dr. Berry emphasizes that blood pH remains stable on a carnivore diet.

## Additional Insights from Other Sources

**Reduced Water Retention:** "Steak and Butter Gal" mentions experiencing a decrease in water weight and fluid retention after transitioning to a carnivore diet. This aligns with Dr. Berry's explanation of diuresis, the increased excretion of water, that occurs as insulin levels normalize.

**Improved Iron Status:** Aaron Edwards, who experienced anemia on a plant-based diet, reports improved hemoglobin, hematocrit, and erythrocyte levels after switching to a carnivore approach, indicating better iron status.

It's crucial to remember that individual responses to a carnivore diet can vary. While these blood work changes are commonly observed, it's essential to consult with a healthcare professional to monitor your health and address any concerns.

# CHAPTER 6

# PLANTS

## Plant PUFAs and Oxidative Stress: A Deep Dive

The sources provide a comprehensive explanation of how polyunsaturated fats (PUFAs) in plants, particularly those found in processed vegetable oils, contribute to oxidative stress. While emphasizing the importance of understanding the nuances of fatty acid metabolism, they offer several key insights.

The sources provide a nuanced and critical perspective on the role of plant PUFAs in promoting oxidative stress. They highlight the importance of moving beyond simplistic views of omega-6s versus omega-3s to focus on the broader issue of PUFA oxidation. They urge readers to critically evaluate dietary guidelines, especially those influenced by financial interests, and prioritize whole food sources of fats and oils to protect their health.

### PUFA Instability and Oxidation

**Double Bonds and Oxygen Reactivity:** PUFAs, both omega-3s and omega-6s, possess multiple double bonds in their chemical structure. These double bonds are highly reactive with oxygen. This reactivity makes PUFAs susceptible to oxidation, a process akin to rusting, where free radicals attack these bonds, causing damage and creating harmful byproducts.

**PUFA Breakdown and Toxin Formation:** When PUFAs oxidize, they break down into harmful compounds, including aldehydes and lipid peroxides. These byproducts are considered toxins that contribute to oxidative stress within the body. The sources emphasize that it's not necessarily the PUFAs themselves that are harmful, but rather their oxidized forms, often referred to as "lipid oxidation products."

## Vegetable Oil Processing and PUFA Vulnerability

**Protective Factors in Whole Foods:** In their natural state within whole plant foods, PUFAs are accompanied by protective antioxidants like vitamin E and other phytonutrients. These antioxidants help stabilize the PUFAs, preventing or slowing down the oxidation process.

Stripping Away Protection: The industrial processing of vegetable oils involves high heat, pressure, and chemical treatments that strip away these protective antioxidants. This processing leaves the PUFAs highly vulnerable to oxidation, both during storage and cooking.

## Consequences of PUFA Oxidation in the Body

**Oxidized LDL and Cardiovascular Risk:** When consumed, oxidized PUFAs from vegetable oils can become incorporated into lipoproteins, particularly LDL cholesterol, often labeled as "bad cholesterol." This oxidation transforms LDL into a vessel for transporting harmful oxidation products throughout the bloodstream, contributing to blood vessel damage and increasing the risk of cardiovascular disease.

**Mitochondrial Dysfunction and Energy Disruption:** Oxidized PUFAs can also disrupt mitochondrial function. Mitochondria, the energy powerhouses of cells, rely on fatty acids for fuel. However, when exposed to oxidized PUFAs, their energy production capacity is compromised. This disruption contributes to metabolic dysfunction, leading to symptoms like fatigue, sugar cravings, and insulin resistance.

## Beyond Omega-6s: A Broader Understanding

**Focusing on Oxidative Stress, Not Just Linoleic Acid:** The sources challenge the common focus on linoleic acid, an omega-6 fatty acid, as the primary culprit in PUFA-related health issues. They stress that while linoleic acid can be problematic, the broader issue is the oxidative stress caused by the consumption of any oxidized PUFAs, including omega-3s.

**Canola Oil: A Misleading "Healthy" Option:** The sources point to canola oil as a prime example of this misconception. Often touted as a heart-healthy option due to its omega-3 content, canola oil, like other vegetable oils, undergoes extensive processing that leaves its PUFAs vulnerable to oxidation. This oxidation negates any potential benefits from its omega-3 content and contributes to the overall oxidative stress burden.

## Addressing the AHA Recommendations

**Financial Ties and Misinformation:** The sources raise significant concerns about the American Heart Association's (AHA) recommendations to consume vegetable oils. They point to financial ties with major vegetable oil producers as a potential conflict of interest, suggesting that these financial incentives may have driven the AHA's promotion of vegetable oils as "heart-healthy" despite a lack of robust scientific evidence.

## Practical Takeaways

**Minimize Vegetable Oil Consumption:** The sources consistently advocate for reducing or eliminating vegetable oil consumption to minimize PUFA oxidation and its associated health risks. They emphasize the importance of choosing whole food sources of fats and oils that retain their natural protective antioxidants.

**Prioritizing Slow, Sustainable Weight Loss:** For individuals who have consumed a diet high in vegetable oils, the sources recommend a gradual approach to weight loss. Rapid weight loss can force the body to burn stored PUFAs at an accelerated rate, potentially overwhelming the body's ability to handle the resulting oxidative stress. A slower, more sustainable approach allows for a gradual reduction in PUFA stores while minimizing potential damage.

## Dr. Chaffee's Perspective on Plant Toxins

Dr. Anthony Chaffee contends that plants, as living organisms, possess defense mechanisms to protect themselves from predation, and these defenses often involve toxic chemicals that can be harmful to humans. His viewpoint, as presented in the sources, is rooted in several key arguments:

### 1. Plants and Animals in an Evolutionary Arms Race

**Survival through Poison:** Dr. Chaffee explains that plants, unable to flee or physically defend themselves, rely on chemical warfare to deter herbivores.

**Abundance of Carcinogens:** He cites his own experience in a cancer biology class where he learned about the abundance of carcinogens in common vegetables. For instance, Brussel sprouts were found to contain over 136 identified human carcinogens.

**Evolutionary Adaptation:** He argues that while certain animals have evolved to tolerate specific plant toxins, humans haven't encountered many of these plants throughout our evolutionary history, making us more susceptible to their harmful effects.

### 2. Plant Toxins as a Dose-Dependent Poison

**Toxicity in Common Foods:** Dr. Chaffee provides numerous examples of toxic compounds found in everyday fruits and vegetables, such as cyanide in cassava root and almonds, solanine in potatoes, and oxalates in spinach and chia seeds.

**Quantity Matters:** He emphasizes that while these toxins might not cause immediate, acute reactions in small amounts, consuming them in large quantities, as often encouraged in plant-based diets, can lead to various health problems.

### 3. The Myth of "Safe" Plants

**All Plants are Poisonous:** Dr. Chaffee asserts that all plants are inherently poisonous, but the degree of toxicity varies depending on the plant and the consumer. He refutes the notion that some plants are safe while others aren't.

**Specific Diets in Nature:** He highlights how animals in the wild, particularly herbivores, consume very specific diets, indicating an adaptation to certain plant toxins and an avoidance of others. This selectivity, he argues, underscores the potential dangers of consuming a wide variety of plants without understanding their potential toxicity.

### 4. Debunking the "More Plants Equals Better Health" Argument

**Misleading Studies:** Dr. Chaffee challenges studies that claim better health outcomes with increased fruit and vegetable consumption, arguing they often fail to account for other dietary factors.

**Confounding Variables:** He points out that these studies often don't isolate the effects of plants from other lifestyle factors or dietary components, making it difficult to establish a direct causal link between plant consumption and improved health.

## 5. Hormesis as an Unreliable Justification

**The Concept of Hormesis:** While acknowledging the potential for some plant toxins to exhibit hormesis - a beneficial effect at low doses - Dr. Chaffee expresses skepticism about its practical application.

**Dosage Uncertainty:** He argues that the hormetic dose for most plant toxins remains unknown and varies widely, making it improbable to consistently achieve a beneficial effect through random consumption.

**Multiple Toxins and Interactions:** Dr. Chaffee points out that plants contain a multitude of toxins, making it highly unlikely that all of them would exert a hormetic effect at the same time and in the same quantities.

## 6. The Impact of Plant Toxins on Specific Populations

**Vulnerability of Aboriginal Populations:** Dr. Chaffee cites the increased susceptibility of Aboriginal populations in Australia to chronic diseases like obesity, diabetes, and cancer when consuming a Western diet high in plant-based foods.

**Lack of Evolutionary Adaptation:** He attributes this vulnerability to a lack of historical exposure to agriculture and the associated genetic adaptations that may have helped other populations tolerate certain plant toxins.

## Key Takeaways from Dr. Chaffee's Perspective

- Plants possess a diverse array of chemical defenses that can be harmful to humans, particularly when consumed in large quantities.

- The notion of "safe" and "unsafe" plants is an oversimplification; all plants contain toxins, and their effects depend on the specific plant, the consumer, and the dosage.

- Studies linking increased plant consumption to better health often fail to account for confounding factors and don't provide conclusive evidence of a direct causal relationship.

- While hormesis may exist for some plant toxins, its practical application is questionable due to dosage uncertainties and the complex interactions of multiple toxins.

- Specific populations, such as those with limited historical exposure to agriculture, may be particularly vulnerable to the harmful effects of plant toxins.

It's important to note that Dr. Chaffee's views on plant toxins are part of a broader discussion on the potential benefits and risks associated with different dietary approaches. His arguments, while thought-provoking, warrant further research and critical evaluation within the larger context of nutritional science and human health.

## Potential Downsides of a High-Fiber, Plant-Based Diet

The sources, primarily advocating for carnivore diets, offer several potential drawbacks to consuming a high-fiber, plant-based diet:

### 1. Nutrient Deficiencies

**Essential Nutrients Lacking in Plants:** The sources consistently emphasize that certain vital nutrients are absent in plant-based foods and can only be obtained from animal sources. One source particularly stresses this point, asserting that while plants and fungi lack essential nutrients found in meat, meat provides all necessary components obtainable from plants. Another source underscores this concern, noting that even a short-term plant-based diet can lead to deficiencies in vitamin B12, essential for various bodily functions.

**Bioavailability Issues:** Even when nutrients are present in plants, the sources argue that their bioavailability, the degree to which the body can absorb and utilize them, is often lower compared to animal sources. One source highlights this issue, claiming that the absorption rate of micronutrients from vegetables is "trash" and asserting that consuming pounds of vegetables is required to match the micronutrient content found in ounces of meat, particularly organ meats like liver. Another source further elaborates, pointing out that the bioavailability of iron in high-fiber plant foods is significantly lower than in animal sources.

### 2. Presence of Anti-nutrients and Toxins

**Plant Defense Mechanisms:** The sources argue that plants, unable to flee or physically defend themselves, have evolved a chemical arsenal of anti-nutrients and toxins to deter predators. One source refers to these compounds as "herbicides and pesticides," designed to target consumers and potentially cause harm.

**Specific Examples**: One source lists examples of these plant defenses, stating that brussels sprouts contain 136 known human carcinogens, while mushrooms contain over a hundred. Another source expands on this, listing a range of plant toxins including oxalates, tannins, phytates, and lectins, all potentially harmful to human health.

**Impact on Digestion and Health:** The sources suggest that these anti-nutrients can interfere with nutrient absorption, disrupt gut health, and contribute to various health issues. One source cautions that overconsumption of carbs, a staple in plant-based diets, leads to glycation, oxidation, and cardiovascular disease due to their inflammatory nature. Another source attributes chronic inflammation, bloating, nausea, brain fog, and fatigue to the consumption of plant-based foods. Another source specifically points to oxalates, found in foods like spinach and chia seeds, as contributors to gastrointestinal distress, kidney stones, arthritis, and brain fog.

### 3. Digestive Challenges with Fiber

**Human Inability to Digest Fiber:** The sources contend that humans, lacking a functional cecum, are incapable of breaking down fiber effectively. One source states that "the need for fiber in human diets is a complete fallacy" and that fiber, being the indigestible portion of plant carbohydrates, can cause inflammation, block nutrient absorption, and worsen constipation.

**Negative Effects of Fiber:** One source presents a study where increasing fiber intake led to more stomach pain, bloating, constipation, and anal bleeding, while lowering or eliminating fiber alleviated these issues. This is further emphasized in another source, where the speaker, who experienced severe colon damage attributed to fiber, advocates for reducing fiber intake and suggests that increased bowel movements due to fiber consumption are not necessarily beneficial, emphasizing the importance of healthy, regular bowel movements rather than frequency.

## 4. Sustainability Concerns

**Environmental Impact of Agriculture:** One source briefly touches upon the environmental impact of large-scale agriculture, suggesting that it deviates significantly from natural food production and can be detrimental.

**Ethical Considerations:** While not explicitly stated in this context, the sources generally advocate for a meat-centric diet, implying an ethical perspective that may view plant-based agriculture as less sustainable or potentially harmful to ecosystems.

## 5. Potential for Boredom and Restrictive Nature

**Limited Food Choices:** Some individuals might find a strict carnivore diet boring due to limited food choices. Although it suggests ways to vary meat preparation and consumption, the inherent restrictive nature of a purely animal-based diet is evident.

*It's crucial to remember that these sources present a particular viewpoint advocating for carnivore diets. While the points raised regarding potential downsides of high-fiber, plant-based diets merit consideration, they may not represent a comprehensive or universally accepted perspective.*

It's essential to:

- **Consult with Healthcare Professionals:** If considering significant dietary changes, consult with a qualified healthcare professional to assess individual needs and potential risks.

- **Consider Individual Variability:** Human responses to diet vary greatly. What works well for one person may not be suitable for another.

- **Explore Diverse Perspectives:** Seeking information from a variety of sources and scientific perspectives is critical for forming a balanced understanding of this complex and often debated topic.

## Plant Sterols: A Hidden Danger?

While plant sterols are often marketed for their cholesterol-lowering effects, the sources present a concerning perspective, suggesting that these compounds may actually pose significant risks to cardiovascular health. This perspective challenges the conventional wisdom surrounding plant sterols and calls for a closer examination of their potential impact on the human body.

### Plant Sterols: Mimicking Cholesterol with Disastrous Consequences

The sources argue that plant sterols, structurally similar to cholesterol, can interfere with essential cholesterol-dependent processes, leading to detrimental health outcomes. This interference arises from the inability of the body to effectively utilize plant sterols, despite their absorption into the bloodstream.

**Disrupting Cholesterol Functions:** Plant sterols, upon entering the body, compete with cholesterol for absorption and utilization. However, subtle molecular differences prevent them from fulfilling the vital roles that cholesterol plays in cell membrane structure, hormone synthesis, and other critical physiological functions.

One source refers to plant sterols as "fake plant cholesterol," highlighting their ability to mimic cholesterol without providing the necessary functionality. This mimicry leads to a disruption of normal physiological processes, potentially compromising cellular health and overall well-being.

**The Paradox of Cholesterol Lowering:** Plant sterols are often lauded for their ability to lower LDL cholesterol levels, a factor traditionally associated with cardiovascular risk. However, the sources challenge this association, suggesting that artificially lowering LDL levels through plant sterol consumption may not translate to improved cardiovascular health.

One source notes that plant sterols interfere with the synthesis of lipoproteins, including LDL, leading to a reduction in circulating cholesterol levels. However, the source questions whether this reduction is truly beneficial, given the essential roles that cholesterol plays in the body.

**Sitosterolemia: A Case Study in Plant Sterol Toxicity**

The sources point to sitosterolemia, a rare genetic disorder characterized by excessive plant sterol absorption, as compelling evidence for the potential dangers of plant sterols. Individuals with this condition experience severe premature atherosclerosis, highlighting the detrimental impact of plant sterol accumulation on cardiovascular health.

One sSource explains that sitosterolemia provides a stark illustration of what can happen when plant sterols are absorbed in unusually high amounts. The severe cardiovascular complications observed in these individuals suggest that even seemingly beneficial effects, such as LDL lowering, may come at a hidden cost.

**Vegetable Oils: A Major Source of Plant Sterols**

The sources emphasize that vegetable oils, widely consumed in the modern diet, are a significant source of plant sterols. This finding raises concerns about the potential contribution of these oils to the overall plant sterol burden in the body.

**Seed Oils and Plant Sterol Concentration:** The sources highlight that seed oils, extracted from plants like soybeans, corn, and canola, contain high concentrations of plant sterols. This concentration stems from the nature of seeds, which utilize sterols for growth and development.

One s notes that while plant sterols are present in various plant foods, seed oils stand out as a particularly rich source. This observation underscores the potential for vegetable oil consumption to significantly increase plant sterol intake.

**Rethinking the Role of Cholesterol in Heart Health**

The sources challenge the long-held belief that high cholesterol is the primary culprit in heart disease. They argue that this view, heavily influenced by the vegetable oil industry, has led to the widespread adoption of cholesterol-lowering strategies that may be doing more harm than good.

**Challenging the Cholesterol Hypothesis:** The sources present evidence suggesting that the relationship between cholesterol and heart disease is more complex than traditionally portrayed. They argue that focusing solely on lowering cholesterol levels may overlook other crucial factors contributing to cardiovascular risk, such as inflammation and oxidative stress.

One source reveals the role of the vegetable oil industry in shaping the narrative around cholesterol. The source explains that the American Heart Association's promotion of vegetable oils and demonization of saturated fat were driven by financial interests, leading to decades of potentially misleading dietary advice.

Another source further challenges the notion that saturated fat raises LDL cholesterol, citing research demonstrating that coconut oil, rich in saturated fat, actually lowered LDL levels. The source proposes that plant sterols in vegetable oils may artificially suppress LDL levels, masking the body's natural cholesterol balance and potentially creating a false sense of security.

**A Need for Further Investigation**

The sources raise important questions about the safety and efficacy of plant sterol consumption, particularly in the context of a diet high in vegetable oils. While further research is needed to fully elucidate the complex interplay between plant sterols, cholesterol, and cardiovascular health, the evidence presented warrants a critical re-evaluation of current dietary recommendations.

## Plant-Based Diets and Male Reproductive Health: A Look at Testosterone and Sperm Production

The sources offer limited direct information on the impact of plant-based diets on testosterone and sperm production. However, some insights can be gleaned from the available information.

**Low-Fat Diets and Testosterone:** One source mentions that low-fat diets in men can lead to decreased testosterone and sperm production, including motility. While not explicitly mentioning plant-based diets, many plant-based diets are inherently low in fat. This suggests a potential link between plant-based eating patterns and reduced testosterone levels.

**Nutrient Deficiencies and Reproductive Health:** The sources highlight the potential for nutrient deficiencies on plant-based diets, specifically mentioning vitamin B12. One source states that vitamin B12 deficiency in women can negatively affect their ability to carry a fetus to full term. While not directly addressing sperm production, it illustrates the importance of adequate nutrition for reproductive health.

**The Importance of Cholesterol:** The sources emphasize the crucial role of cholesterol in hormone production, including testosterone. One source explicitly states that the body makes testosterone from cholesterol. Many plant-based diets are designed to lower cholesterol, which could indirectly affect testosterone production.

**Indirect Implications:** While not directly addressed, the sources' discussion of plant toxins and anti-nutrients raises questions about the potential impact of these compounds on hormonal balance and reproductive health. More research is needed to understand if and how these factors might influence testosterone and sperm production.

It's important to note that the sources primarily focus on the benefits of carnivore diets and the potential downsides of plant-based diets, particularly those high in processed foods and seed oils. More balanced research is needed to fully understand the nuanced effects of various plant-based eating patterns on male reproductive health.

## The Potential Harms of Fruit: A Critical Examination

While fruits are often touted for their health benefits, the sources raise several concerns about their potential harms. These concerns center around the high sugar content, particularly fructose, and the presence of antinutrients and pesticides.

### Sugar: A Hidden Danger Lurking in Fruit?

The sources argue that the high sugar content of fruit, specifically fructose, can contribute to various health issues. This perspective challenges the common view of fruit as a healthy and essential part of a balanced diet.

**Fructose:** More Glycating Than Glucose: Source 15 reveals that fructose is 8-10 times more glycating than glucose. Glycation, a process in which sugar molecules attach to proteins and lipids, is implicated in aging and cellular dysfunction. One source emphasizes the harmful effects of advanced glycation end products (AGEs), believed to be major culprits in both cellular and tissue aging and dysfunction.

**The Hidden Danger of Fructose:** Another source warns about the hidden danger of fructose in fruit and honey because it is not detected by the standard hemoglobin A1c test, which only measures glucose-related glycation. This means individuals consuming high amounts of fructose may have significant glycation damage that goes undetected.

**Fruit as an Evolutionary Adaptation:** Yes another source suggests that the body's ability to store sugar, including fructose, was likely an evolutionary adaptation for survival during times of scarcity. However, in today's environment of abundant and readily available sugary foods, this adaptation may be contributing to metabolic disorders.

**Fruit's Impact on Blood Sugar:** One source highlights the blood sugar-spiking effects of fruit, comparing a modern apple to a "big ball of sugar" due to selective breeding that has increased its sugar content.

**Addiction and Cravings: That same** source discusses the addictive nature of sugar and the challenges of moderation for those struggling with sugar addiction. Another source echoes this sentiment, acknowledging that fruit cravings stem from the brain's desire for the sweet taste.

**Beyond Sugar: Other Concerns About Fruit**

The sources also express concerns about aspects of fruit consumption beyond their sugar content.

**Pesticides and Herbicides:** One source highlights the pervasive presence of pesticides and herbicides in fruits and vegetables, emphasizing that washing does not eliminate these toxins. Source 53 underscores the high pesticide levels found in conventionally grown strawberries.

**Nutrient Deficiency in Modern Fruit:** Another source argues that modern fruits are significantly less nutrient-dense than those grown decades ago due to soil depletion caused by industrial agriculture practices. The source states that an orange today has only 1/17th of the nutrients it would have had 50 years ago.

**Oxalates and Hormonal Disruption:** Yet another source mentions the presence of oxalates in vegetables, which can cause various health issues, and phytoestrogens, which can disrupt hormones. While the source focuses on vegetables, some fruits also contain oxalates, raising potential concerns.

**The "Frankenfruit" Phenomenon:** Some sources criticize the genetic manipulation and artificial selection of modern fruits, labeling them "Frankenfruit". This manipulation has resulted in larger, sweeter, and more visually appealing fruits, but potentially at the cost of nutritional value and natural balance.

**Balancing the Benefits and Risks**

While the sources express concerns about the potential harms of fruit, it's essential to acknowledge that they primarily advocate for carnivore diets. More balanced research is needed to fully understand the nuanced effects of fruit consumption on human health.

**Some points to consider:**

**Type and Quantity Matter:** The sources primarily focus on the negative impacts of modern, highly cultivated, and often processed fruits. The impact of consuming moderate amounts of whole, seasonal, and locally grown fruits may differ.

**Individual Variability:** Sensitivity to sugar and tolerance for antinutrients can vary greatly among individuals. Some people may experience adverse effects from fruit consumption, while others may not.

# CHAPTER 7

# SEED OILS

## Seed Oils are harmful

Here are the two main properties of seed oils that make them harmful to the body, according to Dr. Paul Mason, as described in the provided YouTube transcript:

**Oxidation:** Dr. Mason explains that seed oils are prone to oxidation due to their chemical structure. He compares this process to rusting, explaining that free radicals damage fats and proteins in the body. The polyunsaturated bonds found in seed oils, specifically the double bonds between carbon atoms, make them highly reactive and susceptible to oxidation. Consuming these oxidized oils leads to the incorporation of oxidation products into lipoproteins like chylomicrons and LDL cholesterol, effectively turning LDL into "a vehicle to carry oxidation around [the] circulation." This oxidation process contributes to blood vessel damage and is a significant factor in seed oils' harmful effects.

**"Fake Plant Cholesterol":** Dr. Mason introduces the concept of "fake plant cholesterol," referring to plant sterols or phytosterols found in high concentrations in seed and vegetable oils. These compounds, present in all plant foods, mimic cholesterol but cannot be effectively utilized by the body. While the body attempts to use plant sterols for functions typically performed by cholesterol, the subtle molecular variations prevent proper utilization, leading to deficient functions. Dr. Mason points to the ironic use of plant sterols in lowering lipoprotein levels, explaining that they create "defective cholesterol," hindering the synthesis of LDL. He argues that this therapeutic use of plant sterols to lower cholesterol is misguided. Dr. Mason cites the condition "sitosterolemia," where individuals with a genetic predisposition absorb an unusually high amount of plant sterols, leading to "severe premature atherosclerosis." This condition, he argues, demonstrates the danger of plant sterols and contradicts the notion that they are beneficial for cardiovascular health.

---

**The American Heart Association's Vegetable Oil Recommendation:
A Scandal Rooted in Financial Ties and Misinformation**

---

The sources present a critical perspective on the American Heart Association's (AHA) endorsement of vegetable oils, suggesting it to be a scandal with far-reaching consequences for public health.

Overall, the sources paint a picture of a system where financial interests have overridden scientific integrity, leading to the widespread acceptance of harmful dietary guidelines. They argue that the AHA's endorsement of vegetable oils has contributed to the obesity epidemic and skyrocketing healthcare costs.

**Important Note:** While the sources strongly condemn the AHA's recommendations, it's crucial to acknowledge that these perspectives represent one side of a complex debate. Further research and consideration of alternative viewpoints are necessary to form a comprehensive understanding of this issue.

The criticism revolves around two central themes:

**Financial Ties with Proctor & Gamble:** One source directly points to the AHA's financial relationship with Proctor & Gamble, a major manufacturer of vegetable oils, as a key factor influencing their dietary recommendations. This connection raises concerns about potential conflicts of interest and the prioritization of profit over scientific evidence. The source alleges that the AHA began advocating for vegetable oils as "heart-healthy" shortly after receiving funding from

Proctor & Gamble, despite lacking scientific evidence to support this claim.

**Fabricated Evidence and Misinformation:** This source goes further, accusing the AHA of fabricating evidence over several decades to bolster their claim that cholesterol causes heart attacks. This deliberate spread of misinformation, according to the source, has led to widespread adoption of harmful dietary practices and unnecessary reliance on statin drugs, one of the most dangerous drug classes. The source explicitly states that "the pile of evidence [supporting cholesterol's role in heart attacks] is nonsense," highlighting the deliberate nature of the AHA's actions.

Furthermore, the sources consistently emphasize the detrimental health effects of vegetable oils:

**PUFA Oxidation and Oxidative Stress:** The sources consistently highlight the role of polyunsaturated fatty acids (PUFAs) in vegetable oils as a major contributor to oxidative stress.

**Impact on Cholesterol:** While vegetable oils might lower cholesterol levels, the sources argue that this effect is misleading and potentially harmful. They suggest that vegetable oils contribute to the oxidation of LDL particles, making them more likely to build up in arteries and contribute to heart disease.

**Inability to Fuel Mitochondria:** The sources explain that PUFAs from vegetable oils become incorporated into body fat, hindering the mitochondria's ability to utilize them for energy. This metabolic disruption leads to increased sugar cravings, hypoglycemia, weight gain, and insulin resistance.

## Detrimental Effects of Vegetable Oils: A Deep Dive

The sources highlight numerous potential negative consequences of consuming a diet high in vegetable oils, focusing primarily on their contribution to oxidative stress, metabolic dysfunction, and various chronic diseases. They argue that these oils, often touted as healthy alternatives to animal fats, pose a significant threat to human health due to their unique chemical properties and processing methods.

### Oxidative Stress and Cellular Damage

The sources consistently emphasize that vegetable oils are highly susceptible to oxidation, a process that generates harmful free radicals and leads to cellular damage. This susceptibility stems from their high polyunsaturated fatty acid (PUFA) content, which reacts readily with oxygen, especially when exposed to heat, light, and processing.

### PUFAs as Double-Edged Swords

The sources challenge the notion that omega-3 PUFAs, often praised for their anti-inflammatory properties, are inherently beneficial. They argue that both omega-3 and omega-6 PUFAs are vulnerable to oxidation and can become detrimental when consumed in excess or in the presence of oxidative stress.

One source explains that omega-3s, with their multiple double bonds, are even more susceptible to oxidation than omega-6s. This vulnerability, coupled with widespread oxidative stress in the modern diet and lifestyle, leads to the rapid degradation of omega-3s, diminishing their potential benefits and potentially contributing to harmful effects.

**Vegetable Oil Processing and Oxidation**

The sources describe the intensive processing methods used to extract oil from seeds, such as soybeans, corn, and canola, highlighting how these methods contribute to oxidation and the formation of harmful compounds.

One source details the harsh treatments involved, including high temperatures, pressure, and chemical solvents, which damage the fragile PUFA molecules, leading to oxidation and the formation of toxins. This process results in a final product that already contains some toxins, lacks protective antioxidants, and is primed to generate more toxins upon exposure to light and heat during cooking.

Another source further explains that one of the final refining steps, bleaching, creates trans fats, which are known to be highly toxic. These trans fats act as "accelerants," promoting further oxidation and contributing to the overall toxicity of the oil.

**Oxidative Stress and Chronic Disease**

The sources link the consumption of oxidized vegetable oils to a cascade of negative health outcomes, primarily through the generation of oxidative stress, a state of imbalance between free radicals and antioxidants in the body.

One source describes vegetable oils as "oxidative stress in a bottle," highlighting their potential to overwhelm the body's antioxidant defenses and contribute to the development of chronic diseases.

Another source echoes this sentiment, stating that consuming oxidized oils leads to the formation of oxidized lipoproteins, such as LDL cholesterol, which are highly damaging to blood vessels and contribute to atherosclerosis.

## Metabolic Dysfunction and Insulin Resistance

The sources argue that the consumption of vegetable oils can disrupt metabolic processes, leading to insulin resistance, weight gain, and an increased reliance on sugar for energy. This disruption stems from the incorporation of PUFAs into cell membranes, hindering the efficient use of body fat for energy and promoting sugar cravings.

## PUFAs and Mitochondrial Dysfunction

The sources explain that PUFAs, when incorporated into cell membranes, interfere with the function of mitochondria, the cellular powerhouses responsible for energy production. This interference arises from the vulnerability of PUFAs to oxidation within the mitochondria, where oxygen concentrations are high.

One source describes how the oxidation of PUFAs within mitochondria generates oxidative stress and disrupts energy production, leading to cellular dysfunction and an increased demand for sugar as fuel.

Another source provides further evidence, citing experiments demonstrating that mitochondria fed with omega-3 PUFAs experience a more rapid and severe decline in energy production compared to those fed with omega-6 PUFAs, highlighting the particularly detrimental effects of omega-3s in this context.

**The Energy Model of Insulin Resistance**

The sources propose a model of insulin resistance that centers on the disruption of cellular energy production caused by vegetable oil consumption. They argue that when cells cannot efficiently use body fat for fuel due to PUFA-induced mitochondrial dysfunction, they become reliant on sugar, leading to a chronic state of hypoglycemia and an overreliance on glucose.

One source explains that this energy deficit triggers a cascade of hormonal responses, including the release of stress hormones like adrenaline and cortisol, which further elevate blood sugar levels by breaking down muscle tissue through a process called gluconeogenesis.

This constant demand for sugar overwhelms the body's insulin response, leading to insulin resistance, a key driver of metabolic dysfunction and diseases like type 2 diabetes.

**Low-Carb Diets and PUFA Accumulation**

The sources caution against adopting low-carbohydrate or ketogenic diets while still consuming vegetable oils, arguing that this combination can exacerbate the metabolic problems associated with PUFA accumulation.

One source explains that when carbohydrates are restricted and body fat is loaded with PUFAs, the body struggles to meet its energy needs.

This struggle can lead to the breakdown of muscle tissue for fuel, as evidenced by studies showing increased muscle loss in individuals following ketogenic diets high in vegetable oils.

**Long-Term PUFA Clearance and Metabolic Recovery**

The sources acknowledge that clearing accumulated PUFAs from the body is a gradual process that can take years. However, they emphasize that adopting a diet that eliminates vegetable oils and prioritizes healthy fats can significantly improve metabolic health even before complete PUFA clearance.

One source highlights the importance of gradual weight loss to minimize the release of PUFAs into the bloodstream and reduce oxidative stress. The source advocates for a balanced approach, emphasizing the need to consume sufficient protein to protect muscle mass and prioritize healthy fats to support cellular function.

**Additional Concerns**

**Plant Sterols and Cardiovascular Risk: O**ne source introduces the concept of "fake plant cholesterol," referring to plant sterols found in high concentrations in vegetable oils. These sterols, while often touted for their cholesterol-lowering properties, can actually be detrimental to cardiovascular health.

The source explains that plant sterols mimic cholesterol but cannot be effectively utilized by the body. When absorbed in excess, they interfere with cholesterol-dependent processes and contribute to the development of atherosclerosis, as evidenced by the severe cardiovascular complications observed in individuals with

111

sitosterolemia, a condition characterized by excessive plant sterol absorption.

**Cholesterol and Heart Health Redefined:** The sources challenge the conventional view of cholesterol as a primary driver of heart disease, arguing that this perspective is based on flawed research heavily influenced by the vegetable oil industry.

One source reveals that the American Heart Association's promotion of vegetable oils and the demonization of saturated fat were fueled by funding from the vegetable oil industry, leading to decades of misleading research and dietary recommendations.

Another source further debunks the myth that saturated fat raises LDL cholesterol, citing studies demonstrating that coconut oil, which is high in saturated fat, actually lowered LDL levels. The source argues that vegetable oils, through their plant sterol content, artificially lower LDL levels, masking the body's natural cholesterol balance.

## A Call for Awareness and Dietary Change

The sources advocate for increased awareness of the potential dangers of vegetable oils and a shift toward diets that prioritize whole, unprocessed foods and healthy fats. They emphasize that eliminating these oils is a crucial step toward mitigating oxidative stress, restoring metabolic function, and reducing the risk of chronic disease.

## Dr. Cate Shanahan's Case Against Vegetable Oils: A Deep Dive into Oxidative Stress

Dr. Cate Shanahan, a physician and author featured in the sources, presents a compelling argument against vegetable oils, focusing on their detrimental effects on human health. Her argument centers around the concept of oxidative stress, a process that damages cells and tissues due to an imbalance between free radicals and antioxidants.

By understanding Dr. Shanahan's argument, individuals can make more informed decisions about their dietary choices, particularly regarding vegetable oil consumption, and advocate for a more critical and evidence-based approach to nutritional recommendations within the medical and scientific community.

### The Hateful Eight: Identifying the Culprits

Dr. Shanahan identifies a specific group of vegetable oils, which she dubs "The Hateful Eight," as the primary culprits in promoting oxidative stress. These oils include:

- 3 Cs: Corn, Canola, Cottonseed
- 3 Ss: Soy, Sunflower, Safflower
- 2 Others: Rice Bran, Grapeseed

She emphasizes memorizing these oils to effectively identify them on food labels and make informed dietary choices.

**PUFAs: The Root of the Problem**

Dr. Shanahan's argument focuses on the high concentration of polyunsaturated fatty acids (PUFAs) in these oils. While PUFAs are essential fatty acids, meaning our bodies need them but cannot produce them, their structure makes them highly susceptible to oxidation.

- **Double Bonds and Oxidation:** PUFAs contain multiple double bonds in their chemical structure, making them highly reactive with oxygen. This reactivity leads to the formation of harmful oxidation products, also known as toxins, both during the refining process and within the body.

- **Omega-6 vs. Omega-3: A Misleading Focus:** Dr. Shanahan challenges the common emphasis on the ratio of omega-6 to omega-3 PUFAs in discussions about vegetable oil consumption. She argues that both types of PUFAs contribute to oxidative stress due to their shared susceptibility to oxidation, regardless of their ratio.

- **Canola Oil: A Deceptive Marketing Tactic:** Dr. Shanahan specifically calls out canola oil, often marketed as heart-healthy due to its higher omega-3 content, as misleading. She asserts that canola oil is no healthier than other omega-6-rich oils because it still promotes oxidative stress.

**Vegetable Oil Processing: Amplifying the Dangers**

Dr. Shanahan highlights how the industrial processing of vegetable oils exacerbates their harmful effects:

- **Heat and Pressure: Creating Initial Toxins:** The refining process involves high heat and pressure, which initiates the formation of toxins even before the oil reaches the consumer.

- **Refining Steps: A Chemical Assault:** She details the various refining steps, including degumming, dewaxing, washing, centrifuging, and ultrafiltration, which attempt to remove some of the toxins generated during processing. However, these steps cannot eliminate all toxins and may introduce additional harmful compounds.

- **Bleaching: The Trans Fat Factor:** Dr. Shanahan emphasizes that the bleaching step, a common practice in vegetable oil refining, creates trans fats, another group of harmful fatty acids linked to various health issues. She notes that even the most refined oils contain a residual level of trans fats, further contributing to their toxicity.

**The Consequences: Disrupting Metabolic Health**

Dr. Shanahan explains how the consumption of oxidized PUFAs and their byproducts disrupts metabolic health:

- **Antioxidant Depletion:** The toxins generated from oxidized PUFAs deplete the body's antioxidant defenses, leaving cells more vulnerable to damage.

- **Body Fat Toxicity:** These oxidized PUFAs get incorporated into our body fat, making it "toxic" and difficult for our cells to burn effectively for energy. This leads to a reliance on sugar for fuel, contributing to sugar cravings and metabolic dysfunction.

- **Mitochondrial Dysfunction:** The toxins from oxidized PUFAs can damage mitochondria, the energy-producing powerhouses of our cells, further hindering energy production and contributing to metabolic disorders.

**Beyond Individual Health: A Systemic Scandal**

Dr. Shanahan goes beyond the individual health implications of vegetable oils, highlighting a systemic issue within the medical and scientific community:

The American Heart Association (AHA) and Proctor & Gamble: A Conflict of Interest: She exposes the historical relationship between the AHA and Proctor & Gamble, a major producer of vegetable oils, suggesting that this relationship influenced the AHA's promotion of vegetable oils as heart-healthy despite a lack of scientific evidence.

- **Misleading Cholesterol Guidelines:** Dr. Shanahan criticizes the widespread adoption of cholesterol-lowering guidelines based on flawed research, arguing that these guidelines have led to unnecessary fear of dietary cholesterol and the prescription of potentially harmful statin drugs. She emphasizes that vegetable oils, while lowering cholesterol levels, actually contribute to heart disease by oxidizing LDL particles, making them more likely to build up in arteries.

- **The Importance of Informed Decision-Making:** Dr. Shanahan stresses the need for individuals to be informed consumers of health information, questioning conventional wisdom and seeking evidence-based guidance to make empowered choices about their health and well-being.

# CHAPTER 8

# SCIENCE

## The Randle Cycle, Insulin, Glucagon, and Health

The Randle cycle describes how glucose and fatty acids compete to enter the cell. When both are present, fatty acids can enter the cell but block glucose from entering. This is likely a protective mechanism because high glucose levels are toxic. However, the glucose locked out of the cell ends up damaging the endothelium, the lining of the vascular system.

The sources emphasize that the Randle cycle is a significant factor in metabolic health. Understanding this metabolic interplay is crucial for making informed dietary choices that support long-term health and well-being.

### Consequences of the Randle Cycle

- **Increased Insulin Production:** When carbohydrates and meat are eaten together, the insulin to glucagon ratio increases significantly. This occurs because the carbohydrates stimulate insulin production while the presence of fat from the meat prevents glucose from being utilized, leading to a build-up of glucose in the bloodstream and a subsequent surge in insulin.

- **Endothelial Damage and Atherosclerosis:** The glucose that is locked out of the cell due to the Randle cycle damages the endothelium. This damage makes it possible for LDL particles to get stuck to the endothelium, causing plaque build-up and atherosclerosis. Atherosclerosis is a major risk factor for heart attacks.

- **Aggravated by Seed Oils:** The presence of seed oils, which are high in polyunsaturated fatty acids (PUFAs), worsens the effects of the Randle cycle. When PUFAs are incorporated into cell membranes, they increase the cell's susceptibility to oxidative stress. This oxidative stress further disrupts the cell's ability to use glucose efficiently, exacerbating insulin resistance.

**Implications for Overall Health**

Chronic activation of the Randle cycle, due to a diet high in both carbohydrates and fat, can lead to several health problems:

- **Weight Gain:** The high insulin levels promote fat storage, leading to weight gain.
- **Type 2 Diabetes:** Persistent high insulin levels can lead to insulin resistance and eventually type 2 diabetes.
- **Cardiovascular Disease:** Endothelial damage caused by the Randle cycle increases the risk of atherosclerosis and other cardiovascular diseases.

**Mitigating the Effects of the Randle Cycle**

To minimize the negative health impacts of the Randle cycle:

- **Choose One Fuel Source:** It is better to predominantly utilize either glucose or fatty acids for fuel, rather than constantly mixing them.
- **Prioritize Healthy Carbohydrates:** If carbohydrates are consumed, opt for those that are digested slowly, such as beans and less starchy vegetables. These carbohydrates cause a slower rise in blood sugar, reducing the likelihood of triggering the Randle cycle.

- **Minimize Seed Oil Consumption:** Limit the intake of seed oils to reduce oxidative stress and improve the body's ability to utilize glucose effectively.

**Contrasting Digestive Systems:
Carnivores vs. Herbivores**

The sources primarily focus on the carnivore diet and its potential effects on human health, so they don't offer a detailed comparison of carnivore and herbivore digestive systems. However, Dr. Anthony Chaffee provides a comprehensive explanation of these differences.

Dr. Chaffee's video argues that humans, lacking a functional cecum and possessing a highly acidic stomach and relatively short small intestine, are biologically better suited for a carnivore diet.

The distinct differences between carnivore and herbivore digestive tracts highlight their adaptation to specific food sources. Carnivores prioritize efficient meat digestion, while herbivores have evolved complex systems to extract nutrients from plant fibers.

**Teeth and Jaw Motion**

**Carnivores:** Sharp teeth designed for tearing flesh, with limited side-to-side jaw motion. This restricts their ability to grind plant material.

**Herbivores:** Flat teeth with a wide range of side-to-side motion, allowing for efficient grinding and breakdown of fibrous plant matter.

**Stomach**

**Carnivores:** Single-chambered stomach with highly acidic conditions (pH 1-2), crucial for digesting meat and killing bacteria.

**Herbivores:** Can have either single or multi-chambered stomachs (like ruminants), with less acidic conditions (pH around 4). The multi-chambered system assists in the complex process of breaking down plant fiber.

## Small Intestine

**Carnivores:** Relatively short small intestine, about 3-6 times their body length.

**Herbivores:** Significantly longer small intestine, around 10-12 times their body length, providing a larger surface area for absorbing nutrients from plant matter.

## Cecum

**Carnivores:** Lack a cecum. The cecum is a pouch-like structure that houses bacteria essential for fermenting plant fiber, a process carnivores don't require.

**Herbivores:** Possess a well-developed cecum, crucial for breaking down otherwise indigestible plant fiber and extracting energy.

## Large Intestine

**Carnivores:** Short and smooth large intestine.

**Herbivores:** Large and often complex large intestine, accommodating additional fermentation of plant material.

---

**Impact of the Agricultural Revolution on Human Brain Size**

---

The sources generally agree that the Agricultural Revolution, a period marked by a shift from hunter-gatherer lifestyles to farming and settled agriculture, had a negative impact on human brain size.

It's important to note that the relationship between the Agricultural Revolution and human brain size is complex and there is ongoing scientific debate on this topic. The sources present a particular perspective that emphasizes the benefits of a meat-based diet and highlights the potential drawbacks of agriculture. It is recommended to consider these arguments in light of other scientific perspectives and research on human evolution and diet.

**Brain Size Reduction:** One source states that after the transition to agriculture, there was a "sharp decline in... brain size by 11%." This reduction suggests that the dietary and lifestyle changes associated with agriculture may have had detrimental effects on human brain development.

**Shift to Plant-Based Diets:** The sources argue that the Agricultural Revolution led to a significant increase in the consumption of plant-based foods, particularly grains. One source highlights that "around this exact same time," referring to the Agricultural Revolution around 12,000 years ago, "humans did do something a little bit interesting too... [t]his happened around 12,000 years ago which is the agriculture Revolution." It continues to note that with this shift, "[d]iseases and things that didn't originally exist even in humans at all for instance Mal occlusion of the teeth tooth decay inflammation of the gums… did start to exist."

**Nutritional Deficiencies:** The sources propose that the reliance on grains and other cultivated crops may have led to nutritional deficiencies, potentially impacting brain development. Another source emphasizes that "there is absolutely nothing that you have to have nothing there's nothing in plants or fungus that you have to have that you cannot get from meat but there are things in meat that you have to have that you cannot get from plants."

**Increased Disease Burden:** One source notes that the Agricultural Revolution "coincided with all of the disease States as well as malocclusion tooth decay and inflammation of the gums." The increased disease burden associated with agriculture may have also contributed to a decline in overall health and, potentially, brain size.

**Possible Explanations**

While the sources don't explicitly explain the reasons behind the reduction in brain size, the following possibilities are suggested:

**Reduced Nutrient Density:** The sources argue that a diet primarily composed of meat is more nutrient-dense than a plant-based diet. A shift towards agriculture might have led to a lower intake of crucial nutrients for brain development, such as fats and certain vitamins.

**Increased Toxin Exposure:** Cultivated plants, especially grains, may contain anti-nutrients and other toxins that could interfere with nutrient absorption and overall health, potentially affecting brain development.

**Changes in Lifestyle:** The transition to a settled lifestyle might have led to reduced physical activity and mental stimulation, possibly contributing to a decrease in brain size.

## The Carnivore Diet and Testosterone Levels: Insights and Speculation

The sources offer limited direct information about the impact of a carnivore diet on testosterone levels in men and women. However, we can glean some insights and potential connections from the available information, keeping in mind that these are largely speculative and require further research for confirmation.

### Men: Potential for Increased Testosterone

**Cholesterol as a Precursor:** One key factor to consider is that testosterone is synthesized from cholesterol. Source 64 explicitly states that "your body makes testosterone from cholesterol." A carnivore diet, being rich in animal fats, naturally leads to higher cholesterol intake. It's plausible that this increased cholesterol availability could potentially contribute to higher testosterone production in men.

**Anecdotal Evidence:** One source provides a personal account of a man who experienced a significant increase in his testosterone levels after adopting a carnivore diet for six months. His testosterone level more than doubled, going from a low level to well within the normal range. While this is just one individual's experience, it suggests a possible link between a carnivore diet and increased testosterone in men.

### Women: A More Complex Picture

The sources provide even less specific information regarding the impact of a carnivore diet on testosterone levels in women.

126

**Potential for Hormonal Imbalances:** Some sources, while not directly addressing the carnivore diet, raise concerns about the potential for hormonal imbalances in women following restrictive diets, particularly those that severely limit carbohydrate intake.

**Menstrual Irregularities:** One source discusses concerns about menstrual irregularities and potential infertility in women following a carnivore diet. However, the source also presents counter-arguments, highlighting a woman who has successfully followed a carnivore diet for 13 years with seemingly no adverse effects on her health or fertility.

**Importance of Individualized Assessment:** It's crucial to recognize that hormonal responses to dietary changes vary significantly among women. Factors such as age, health status, activity levels, and previous dietary patterns can all play a role. A carnivore diet might affect hormone levels differently in different women.

### General Considerations

**Insulin Sensitivity:** The sources consistently emphasize the role of insulin in regulating various metabolic processes. Source 60 highlights the high prevalence of insulin resistance in the modern population, linking it to various health issues, including hormonal imbalances. A carnivore diet, by promoting insulin sensitivity, could potentially have a positive impact on hormone regulation in both men and women.

**Nutrient Intake:** Adequate intake of essential nutrients is crucial for hormone production and balance. A well-formulated carnivore diet should provide sufficient amounts of nutrients like zinc, magnesium, and vitamin D, all of which play a role in testosterone production.

**Stress and Cortisol:** Chronic stress can negatively impact hormone levels, particularly testosterone. Source 73 links poor sleep, a common stressor, to elevated cortisol levels, which can suppress testosterone production. It's essential to address stress management strategies alongside dietary changes.

**The Need for More Research**

The current evidence regarding the impact of a carnivore diet on testosterone levels is largely anecdotal and speculative. More research is needed to investigate the potential benefits and risks, particularly for women.

It's important to reiterate that the information presented here is based on interpretations of the provided sources and should not be considered medical advice. Consulting with a qualified healthcare professional is essential for making informed dietary choices, especially those involving significant dietary changes.

## The Carnivore Diet and Insulin Levels:
## Insights from the Sources

The sources suggest that a carnivore diet leads to significantly lower and more stable insulin levels compared to diets that include carbohydrates. This effect is attributed to the absence of carbohydrates and the resulting minimal stimulation of insulin release.

**Carbohydrates as the Primary Insulin Stimulator:** The sources consistently emphasize that carbohydrates are the primary dietary trigger for insulin release. One source explains this fundamental concept: "One way we increase blood sugar is by eating foods rich in carbohydrates. Carbohydrates are broken down by the body into glucose, which enters the bloodstream. When blood sugar rises, the pancreas releases insulin."

**Absence of Carbohydrates, Minimal Insulin Response:** A carnivore diet, by eliminating all carbohydrates, essentially removes this primary insulin-stimulating factor. As a result, the pancreas releases very little insulin.

**Metabolic Shift to Fat Adaptation:** The sources explain that when the body is consistently deprived of carbohydrates, it undergoes a metabolic shift towards fat adaptation. In this state, the body becomes highly efficient at utilizing fat as its primary fuel source, further reducing the need for glucose and consequently, insulin.

**Fasting Insulin Reduction:** One source specifically mentions that individuals following a carnivore diet experience a "drastic reduction" in their fasting insulin levels. This finding suggests that the absence of dietary carbohydrates leads to a sustained reduction in insulin production even when not actively eating.

**Potential Benefits of Lower Insulin Levels**

The sources highlight several potential benefits associated with lower and more stable insulin levels, particularly for individuals with metabolic dysfunction or those at risk of developing such conditions:

**Improved Insulin Sensitivity:** Chronically elevated insulin levels can lead to insulin resistance, a condition where the body's cells become less responsive to insulin's signals. One source notes that insulin resistance is a precursor to type 2 diabetes and is highly prevalent in the modern population. The sources suggest that a carnivore diet, by keeping insulin levels low, can help improve insulin sensitivity and potentially reverse insulin resistance.

**Reduced Inflammation:** The sources repeatedly link high insulin levels to chronic inflammation, a key driver of many chronic diseases. By reducing insulin levels, a carnivore diet could potentially contribute to lower inflammation throughout the body.

**Weight Loss:** When insulin levels are chronically elevated, the body tends to store fat rather than burn it. Lowering insulin levels, as achieved through a carnivore diet, shifts the body's metabolism towards fat burning, potentially promoting weight loss.

**Improved Metabolic Health:** The sources present the carnivore diet as a highly effective approach for improving various markers of metabolic health, including blood sugar control, cholesterol levels, and

130

triglyceride levels. These improvements are largely attributed to the diet's impact on insulin levels and insulin sensitivity.

**Potential Challenges and Considerations**

**Adaptive Glucose Sparing:** One source discusses a phenomenon known as "adaptive glucose sparing," which can occur when someone has been on a low-carb diet for an extended period. In this state, the body becomes so efficient at using fat for fuel that even small amounts of carbohydrates can lead to a temporary rise in blood sugar. This effect is not necessarily harmful and may simply reflect the body's adaptation to a low-carbohydrate metabolic state.

**Individual Variability:** It's crucial to acknowledge that individual responses to a carnivore diet, particularly regarding insulin levels and blood sugar regulation, can vary. Factors such as genetics, metabolic health, activity levels, and stress levels can all influence how the body adapts to this dietary approach.

**Key Takeaway**

The sources strongly suggest that a carnivore diet leads to significant reductions in insulin levels due to the elimination of carbohydrates. This effect, coupled with the metabolic shift to fat adaptation, is presented as a major driver of the diet's potential benefits for improving insulin sensitivity, reducing inflammation, promoting weight loss, and enhancing overall metabolic health. However, individual responses may vary, and it's essential to monitor health markers and adjust the diet as needed under the guidance of a qualified healthcare professional.

## The Mongol Diet and Its Contribution to Their Success

The sources provide fascinating insights into how the Mongols' heavily meat-based diet might have contributed to their military dominance and the establishment of their vast empire.

**Mobility and Subsistence:** The sources highlight the Mongols' ability to sustain themselves for extended periods on a diet primarily consisting of meat, blood, and milk from their livestock, particularly horses. Two sources describe how this dietary strategy allowed them to cover vast distances without being burdened by the need for frequent meals or extensive food supplies. Another source elaborates on this point, explaining that the Mongols could travel for days without eating, then consume large quantities of horse meat when available, sustaining them for another extended period. This dietary flexibility, enabled by their carnivorous lifestyle, gave them a significant advantage in warfare, allowing for rapid movement and sustained campaigns across vast and often unforgiving terrains.

**Nutritional Advantages for Warfare:** The sources suggest that the Mongols' meat-heavy diet provided them with physical and mental advantages that contributed to their military prowess. One source describes how Mongol warriors would often consume horse blood, a practice also observed in the Samburu tribe of Africa, suggesting that this practice provided them with essential nutrients and energy. While consuming blood might seem unusual from a modern perspective, it likely offered a readily available source of iron and other vital nutrients that could have contributed to their endurance and resilience in battle.

**Psychological Impact:** The sources portray the Mongols as a formidable and even fearsome force, and their dietary practices likely played a role in shaping this image. The Mongols were known for their physical strength and dominance, and their diet, rich in protein and fat from animal sources, could have contributed to their muscular builds and overall robustness. This perception of the Mongols as physically powerful and capable warriors, fueled by their meat-centered diet, could have had a psychological impact on their enemies, contributing to a sense of intimidation and potentially influencing the outcome of battles.

It's important to note that while the sources strongly emphasize the role of the Mongols' meat-based diet in their success, other factors undoubtedly played a significant role in their military achievements, such as their superior horsemanship, military tactics, and organizational skills. Additionally, while the Mongols primarily consumed animal products, their diet might have included some plant-based foods when available, particularly during times of scarcity or when conquering regions with more diverse food resources.

In summary, the sources paint a compelling picture of how the Mongols' unique dietary practices, centered around animal products, might have played a crucial role in their military successes. Their ability to subsist on a meat-heavy diet provided them with logistical advantages, potentially enhanced their physical and mental capabilities, and likely contributed to their formidable reputation as a dominant force in history.

## Rethinking Cholesterol: Insights from the Sources

The sources present a perspective that challenges conventional thinking about cholesterol, suggesting that it might not be the health villain it's often portrayed to be.

**Cholesterol as a Fundamental Building Block:** The sources emphasize the vital role cholesterol plays in the body. One source underscores that cholesterol is the precursor to "all the hormones that you're probably thinking of," highlighting its essentiality for hormone production. This perspective suggests that maintaining adequate cholesterol levels is crucial for overall health and hormonal balance.

**Questioning the LDL Focus:** The sources challenge the common practice of solely focusing on LDL cholesterol levels as a measure of cardiovascular health. One source argues that "the LDL number is not the number that one should be harping over," suggesting that other factors, such as inflammation and insulin resistance, might be more relevant indicators of heart disease risk. Another source echoes this sentiment, urging individuals to consider a broader picture of health, including overall well-being and other blood markers, rather than fixating solely on LDL cholesterol.

**Distinguishing Between Oxidized and Un-oxidized LDL:** The sources highlight the importance of understanding the difference between oxidized and un-oxidized LDL cholesterol. One source emphasizes that while regular LDL cholesterol, even at elevated levels, doesn't necessarily contribute to plaque buildup in arteries, oxidized LDL is the real culprit. This perspective suggests that reducing oxidative stress, rather than simply lowering LDL cholesterol, should be a primary focus for heart health. Another source further reinforces this point, stating that oxidized LDL, regardless of its concentration, "does build up in Our arteries" and can contribute to heart disease.

**Shifting the Focus from Cholesterol to Root Causes:** The sources suggest that addressing the root causes of heart disease, such as inflammation and insulin resistance, is more effective than solely focusing on lowering cholesterol levels. One source argues that "vegetable oils probably cause heart attacks" by promoting oxidative stress and inflammation, suggesting that dietary choices play a significant role in cardiovascular health. Another source emphatically states that "neither cholesterol [nor] saturated fat cause heart disease," implying that other factors, such as processed food consumption and unhealthy lifestyle choices, might be the primary drivers of heart problems.

**Dietary Strategies to Reduce Oxidative Stress**

The sources recommend dietary interventions to mitigate oxidative stress and promote heart health.

**Eliminating Seed Oils:** The sources consistently emphasize the importance of avoiding seed oils, which they claim contribute significantly to oxidative stress and inflammation. One source labels seed oils as "absolutely deleterious to the human body" due to their high concentration of polyunsaturated fats, which are prone to oxidation. Another source asserts that eliminating seed oils from the diet is crucial for reducing oxidized LDL and improving cardiovascular health.

**Adopting a Carnivore or Low-Carbohydrate Diet:** The sources suggest that a carnivore or low-carbohydrate diet, which prioritizes animal-based foods and minimizes processed foods and sugars, can be beneficial for reducing inflammation and improving metabolic health. One source highlights the potential of a low-carbohydrate diet to lower insulin levels and improve insulin sensitivity, factors often linked to heart disease.

It's important to note that while the sources offer compelling arguments against the conventional fear of cholesterol, they represent a specific perspective within the broader scientific and medical community. Consulting with a healthcare professional to discuss individual health concerns and appropriate dietary choices is always recommended.

## Fiber: Essential or Overblown?

The sources you've provided present a perspective that challenges the widely held belief that fiber is essential for human health, particularly for digestion.

**Humans Can Thrive Without Fiber:** Several sources directly assert that the human body can function effectively without dietary fiber. One source claims, "The need for fiber in human diets is a complete fallacy," arguing that all carbohydrates, including fiber, are non-essential for humans. Another source goes further, stating that, except for breast milk during infancy, "human beings do not need a carbohydrate to pass their lips their entire life," implying that fiber is unnecessary at any stage of life.

**Fiber's Negative Impact on Nutrient Absorption:** Some sources argue that fiber can actually hinder nutrient absorption. One source cites a 1978 study comparing high-fiber to low-fiber diets. The study found that high-fiber diets resulted in "more than a doubling of the nutrition that was lost into the feces," meaning that essential nutrients were not absorbed properly and were excreted instead. Another source further suggests that fiber, along with lectins and phytic acids found in plant foods, "can block...co-actors" like zinc and various B vitamins "by as much as 100%," further hindering nutrient absorption. This perspective challenges the common belief that fiber aids digestion and nutrient uptake, suggesting instead that it might have a detrimental effect.

Fiber as a Potential Irritant to the Gut: Several sources claim that fiber can be a source of irritation and discomfort in the gut, contrary to the common belief that it promotes regularity and digestive health. Source 2 describes fiber as "toxic" and "destructive to your anic function," claiming that it can be "pro-inflammatory" and ultimately compromise health. Source 17 expands on this, explaining that fiber, being indigestible, adds bulk to stool, potentially leading to constipation. It also notes that the fermentation of fiber by gut bacteria can produce methane gas, causing bloating and discomfort. Yet another source further emphasizes the potential negative impact of fiber on gut health, stating that consuming plants, particularly those high in fiber, caused their ostomy bag to "blow up like a balloon." This personal experience, while anecdotal, reinforces the idea that fiber might not be as beneficial for gut health as conventionally promoted.

**Nutritional Ketosis as a Superior Alternative to Fiber for Colon Health:** One source ntroduces the concept of nutritional ketosis as a potentially more effective way to nourish the cells lining the colon (colonocytes) than relying on fiber fermentation. It argues that while fiber fermentation produces short-chain fatty acids that are converted into ketones to nourish colonocytes, nutritional ketosis directly provides ketones in the bloodstream, benefiting all cells, including those in the colon. This perspective suggests that a low-carbohydrate, high-fat diet that induces nutritional ketosis might be a superior approach to supporting colon health compared to consuming fiber.

**Addressing Constipation Without Fiber:** The sources acknowledge that constipation is a common concern for those considering a low-fiber or carnivore diet. However, they offer alternative solutions for addressing this issue. One source suggests that increasing fat intake on a carnivore diet can help regulate bowel movements and alleviate constipation. Another source, based on personal experience, advocates for a meat-heavy diet for optimal digestion, claiming that "everything that you are eating is easily absorbed" on a carnivore diet, resulting in less frequent bowel movements without constipation. This contradicts the conventional advice to increase fiber intake for regularity, suggesting that a low-fiber approach can be effective for maintaining healthy bowel function.

**Reframing the Narrative on Fiber:** The sources collectively challenge the dominant narrative surrounding fiber, suggesting that its importance for human health might be overblown. They argue that fiber is not essential, can hinder nutrient absorption, and may even be detrimental to gut health in some cases. Instead, they propose alternative approaches to digestive health, such as focusing on fat intake and embracing nutritional ketosis.

While the sources present a compelling case against the necessity of fiber, it's essential to remember that they represent a particular perspective. Consulting with a healthcare professional to discuss individual health concerns and appropriate dietary choices is always advisable.

## The Gut Microbiome:
## A Complex Ecosystem with Profound Implications

The sources provide insights into the role of the gut microbiome in human health, particularly emphasizing the impact of diet and the potential for dysfunction caused by modern dietary practices.

While the sources offer a compelling perspective on the significance of the gut microbiome and its impact on health, it's important to remember that this field of research is still evolving. Consulting with a healthcare professional to discuss individual health concerns and appropriate dietary choices is always recommended.

### The Microbiome as a Key Player in Digestion and Nutrient Absorption

The sources highlight that the bacteria residing in our gut play a crucial role in digesting food and making nutrients available to our bodies.

One source emphasizes this point, stating, "Most of us don't realize that we don't digest our own food, the bacteria do." This perspective challenges the notion that our bodies solely process food, highlighting the collaborative relationship between humans and their gut microbiome.

Another source, in our conversation history, supports this idea by stating that high-fiber diets can increase nutrient loss in feces, suggesting that fiber might interfere with the gut microbiome's ability to efficiently extract nutrients.

**The Influence of Diet on Microbiome Composition and Function**

The sources underscore that the types of food we consume directly impact the composition and activity of our gut microbiome.

One source emphasizes this concept, stating that "healthy bacteria only survive on protein and fat," while "harmful pathogenic bacteria...thrive on starches and sugars." This perspective suggests that a diet rich in animal-based foods might support a beneficial bacterial balance, while a diet high in processed foods and carbohydrates could promote the growth of harmful bacteria. This aligns with the sources' overall advocacy for a carnivore or low-carbohydrate diet for optimal health.

**The Gut-Brain Connection and Mental Health**

The sources emphasize the intricate connection between the gut microbiome and the brain, highlighting the potential impact of gut health on mental well-being.

One source stresses the significance of this connection, stating, "That gut is so central to what's going on in our minds and in our bodies." This perspective underscores the importance of maintaining a healthy gut microbiome for optimal mental and emotional function.

Another source, in our conversation history, supports this notion by noting that studies have found a correlation between vegan and vegetarian diets and an increased prevalence of mental health issues. This suggests that dietary choices can influence the gut microbiome, which, in turn, can impact mental health.

## The Microbiome's Role in Immune System Development and Function

One source explicitly states that "the microbiome is actually what builds our immune system." This perspective highlights the crucial role of the gut microbiome in training and supporting our immune defenses, emphasizing its importance in protecting us from disease.

## Potential for Microbiome Imbalances and Health Consequences

The sources emphasize that imbalances in the gut microbiome, often caused by modern dietary practices, can contribute to various health problems. One source highlights that chronic illness, stress, and consumption of sugary processed foods can "kill your healthy bacteria," leading to an overgrowth of harmful bacteria. This perspective suggests that modern lifestyle factors can disrupt the delicate balance of the gut microbiome, potentially leading to a cascade of negative health outcomes.

## Restoring Gut Health Through Dietary Interventions

The sources suggest that adopting a diet focused on whole, unprocessed foods, particularly animal-based foods, can help restore a healthy gut microbiome. One source highlights that "killing off the bacteria...getting that back to symbiosis" can be achieved through dietary changes. This perspective aligns with the sources' overall advocacy for a carnivore or low-carbohydrate diet as a means of promoting gut health and, consequently, overall well-being.

# THE SOURCES

---

**Source #1**

**9 Painful Lessons You'll Learn Starting Carnivore**

---

The video by "Steak and Butter Gal." aims to guide new carnivore dieters through the challenges they might encounter while adjusting to this restrictive lifestyle.

The video is structured around nine common struggles experienced by carnivore dieters, each presented as a "painful lesson." These include feeling isolated, facing societal judgment, finding it difficult to socialize, not seeing immediate progress, developing meat aversion, experiencing carb withdrawal symptoms, dealing with oxalate dumping, adjusting to bowel changes, and battling cravings.

For each lesson, the creator offers actionable steps and solutions, drawing on her own personal experience as a long-time carnivore dieter.

Ultimately, the video serves to provide support, encouragement, and practical advice to help viewers overcome the hurdles and successfully adopt the carnivore diet.

---

*https://youtu.be/*a4dZxRz4Iao

---

**Key Sections and Arguments**

**Stool Changes:** This section addresses common digestive issues faced when transitioning to a carnivore diet. It suggests reducing fat intake for diarrhea and increasing salt and fat for constipation.

144

**Craving Management:** This section offers strategies for managing cravings, including removing temptations from your environment and reinforcing your motivation for adopting the diet.

---

**Source #2**

**BEN BIKMAN mcB7 | PLANTS: MEN:**

**lower T, sperm WOMEN: no B12**

---

The video discusses the effects of plant-based diets, artificial sweeteners, and diet sodas on insulin levels.

Dr. Birkman argues that while plant-based diets can reduce insulin resistance due to calorie restriction, they can also lead to nutrient deficiencies, particularly in B12. He criticizes plant-based diets for potentially harming human health, citing negative effects on testosterone and sperm production in men and fetal development in women.

He also asserts that allulose, an artificial sweetener, does not stimulate insulin production, making it a healthier alternative to other sweeteners, like Stevia or monk fruit extract. However, Dr. Birkman acknowledges that artificial sweeteners like aspartame in diet sodas do not directly raise insulin levels, but they may lead to an increase in snacking and hunger, ultimately contributing to weight gain.

Dr. Birkman advises against diet sodas if they trigger excessive snacking or cravings.

---

*https://youtu.be/A5TEjpICmhA*

---

> ## Source #3
> ## Bart Kay Debunks Diet Myths:
> ## What Your Nutrition Guru Won't Tell You

This is a conversation between Bart Kay, a proponent of the carnivore diet, and an individual who has undergone an ostomy surgery. The conversation focuses on debunking diet myths and advocating for a purely meat-based diet for optimal human health.

- Kay argues that the human body is best adapted to consuming meat and fat, asserting that our ancestors primarily consumed animal products and minimal plant material.
- Kay claims that plant-based foods, particularly those cultivated for modern consumption, contain toxins and anti-nutrients that can cause various health problems.
- Kay emphasizes that consuming carbohydrates and sugar, even in the form of honey or fruit, can lead to negative health outcomes like glycation and insulin resistance.

Kay concludes by stating that humans are not designed to consume large quantities of carbohydrates and that a strictly meat-based diet is the most natural and beneficial way to live.

> *https://youtu.be/S9Bu-r3KEbk*

**Key Sections and Arguments**

**Medical Misinformation and Plant-Based Diets:** This section critiques the lack of adequate nutrition education in medical training

147

and argues that plant-based diets can harm gut health and lead to conditions like ostomy surgery.

**Carbohydrates, Sugar, and Diabetes:** This excerpt emphasizes the detrimental effects of excessive sugar consumption, arguing that it contributes to diabetes and contradicts the natural human diet of meat and fat.

---

**Source #4**

**Botany 101: Plant Toxins in Your Daily Diet &**
**Why You Need to Know!**

---

In this YouTube video, Dr. Anthony Chaffee talks about plant toxins and their potential impact on human health. Dr. Chaffee, a doctor, argues that plants, as living organisms, produce toxins to protect themselves from predators.

- Dr. Chaffee highlights that most plants contain a variety of toxins, including carcinogens, and that these toxins can cause a range of health issues, from acute poisoning to long-term effects like cancer.
- Dr. Chaffee advocates for a primarily meat-based diet, claiming that avoiding plant-based foods has significantly improved his health.
- He also mentions that some animals, such as koalas and pandas, have evolved to digest specific plants, but ingesting other plant species can make them sick.

The video ends with a discussion about the abundance of toxins in various plants, including fruits and mushrooms, and encourages viewers to consider the potential risks of consuming them.

---

*https://youtu.be/uMahgg9tVUc*

---

**Key Sections and Arguments**

**The Prevalence of Plant Toxins and Their Health Effects:** This section explores the wide variety of plant toxins present in commonly consumed foods, highlighting their potential for causing acute poisoning, allergic reactions, and long-term consequences like cancer and damage to various organ systems.

**The Dangers of Mushrooms and Cyanogenic Glycosides:** This excerpt provides specific examples of plant toxins, such as those found in poisonous mushrooms and cassava root, emphasizing the need for careful preparation and awareness of potential risks.

**The Impact of Plant Toxins on Mitochondria and Cancer:** This section connects plant toxins to mitochondrial damage and cancer development, emphasizing the role of carcinogens in disrupting cellular processes and contributing to disease.

**Source #5**
**CHEAT On Carnivore? The Gut Truth You Need to Know!**

This video discusses the connection between the microbiome, diet, and overall health, specifically focusing on the benefits of a 100% carnivore diet.

The speaker, Malia, shares her personal journey with chronic illness and how adopting a carnivore diet, rich in protein and fat, helped her overcome debilitating anxiety, depression, and other health issues. She emphasizes the crucial role of healthy gut bacteria in digestion, immune function, and even mental well-being.

Malia highlights the Integrated Health Foundation's (IHF) program, which focuses on addressing chronic illness through a combination of dietary changes, lifestyle modifications, and limbic system rewiring.

The video aims to raise awareness about the importance of the microbiome and advocate for a more holistic approach to health, encouraging viewers to explore the potential benefits of a carnivore diet and the IHF's program.

*https://youtu.be/QSNAz0zcads*

---

**Source #6**
**Carnivore Diet will do this to Your Labs**
**[Carnivore Diet Results]- 2024**

---

This YouTube video by Dr. Ken Berry, a family physician, discusses the potential effects of a carnivore diet on various blood tests. Dr. Berry emphasizes that a carnivore diet, consisting solely of animal products like meat, eggs, and seafood, can lead to significant improvements in lab results, especially after three months.

Dr. Berry outlines how the diet can impact blood counts, liver and kidney function, cholesterol levels, blood sugar, insulin levels, hormones, inflammation markers, and thyroid function.

Notably, he debunks the common misconception that eating meat increases blood acidity, asserting that a carnivore diet actually helps regulate blood pH and has numerous health benefits, such as reversing type 2 diabetes, reducing fatty liver, and improving hormonal balance.

Dr. Berry encourages viewers to get their blood tests checked before and after embarking on a carnivore diet to monitor these potential changes.

---

*https://youtu.be/2endHpgD00A*

---

**Key Sections and Arguments**

**Long-Term Benefits and Elimination of Vices:** This excerpt showcases the long-term positive impacts of the carnivore diet, including the natural reduction of cravings and the disappearance of unhealthy habits.

**Willpower vs. Hormonal Balance:** This section argues against relying solely on willpower for dietary success, emphasizing the crucial role of hormonal balance achieved through the carnivore diet.

**Taste Changes and Satiety Cues:** This excerpt describes the subtle taste changes and heightened satiety experienced on a carnivore diet, highlighting the unique satisfaction derived from each meal.

**Diet Soda and Headache Relief:** This section presents anecdotal evidence suggesting a connection between diet soda consumption and headaches, advocating for its elimination.

**The Speaker's Background and Expertise:** This excerpt details the speaker's professional journey and qualifications, establishing their credibility as an Oral Facial Pain specialist and advocate for the carnivore diet.

**Source #7**

**Doctor Explains: Why Hormones Love Carnivore**

This excerpt is a conversation between Dr. Eric Grin, a specialist in Oral Facial Pain, and Dave, a well-known figure in the carnivore diet community. Dr. Grin shares his compelling personal experience with adopting a carnivore diet, highlighting the significant weight loss, improved satiety, and reduction of cravings he experienced.

Dr. Grin emphasizes that this dietary approach is not about willpower but about realigning one's hormones to achieve true satiety and ultimately achieve health goals.

Dr. Grin, being a medical professional, also delves into the issue of association versus causation, particularly within the context of nutrition science, underscoring the need for rigorous research and caution against drawing conclusions based on mere correlation.

He argues that the medical community often overlooks the importance of a whole-food diet, perpetuating unhealthy habits that lead to widespread chronic diseases like obesity and diabetes.

Dr. Grin concludes by expressing his hope for a greater awareness of the negative impact of processed foods and a shift towards a more holistic approach to health.

*https://youtu.be/QiksUyd71Gs*

---

**Source #8**

**Dr Ken Berry: The Carnivore Beginner Guide (2024 - Updated)**

---

This podcast interview with Dr. Ken Berry, a physician who advocates for the carnivore diet focuses on Dr. Berry's personal experience with the carnivore diet, its benefits and how to get started.

The interview also addresses common misconceptions about the carnivore diet and its potential risks.

Dr. Berry emphasizes that the carnivore diet is a natural and ancestrally appropriate way of eating, which has significantly improved his health and well-being.

He encourages listeners to try the carnivore diet for 90 days to experience its benefits for themselves.

---

*https://youtu.be/bxgjPOr7GEs*

---

**Key Sections and Arguments**

**Evolutionary Basis for Carnivore:** This excerpt establishes the evolutionary foundation for the carnivore diet, emphasizing the historical consumption of meat and fat by homo sapiens.

**Intuitive Eating and Salt Consumption:** This section advocates for intuitive eating on the carnivore diet, allowing for self-regulation of food intake and salt consumption based on individual needs and taste preferences.

**The Importance of Salt:** This excerpt stresses the importance of salt as an essential nutrient, drawing parallels with animals' natural instinct to seek it out.

**Water and Coffee Consumption on Carnivore:** This section discusses the consumption of water and black coffee on a carnivore diet, suggesting mineral supplementation to mimic naturally occurring mineral-rich water.

**Community Impact and Personal Responsibility:** This excerpt emphasizes the potential of individual health transformations to inspire positive change in communities.

**Food Choices and Honoring Your Body:** This section contrasts processed foods with real food, advocating for prioritizing the latter and honoring your body through mindful food choices.

**The Author's Platform and Resources:** This excerpt introduces Dr. Ken Berry's various platforms and resources, including his YouTube channel, social media presence, and published books, highlighting his role as a prominent voice in the carnivore community.

---

**Source #9**
**Dr Leslyn Keith: High-Fat Carnivore Diet**
**Shows Spectacular Results**

---

This is an interview with Dr. Leslyn Keith, a lymphatic therapist who promotes the use of a ketogenic, or even carnivore, diet for the treatment of lymphatic disorders.

Dr. Keith explains how she originally began exploring these types of diets as a way to help her patients lose weight, but soon discovered that they had a profound effect on the lymphatic system itself.

She emphasizes that a high-carb diet is inflammatory to the lymphatic system, whereas fat and ketones are readily utilized and even promote the growth of new lymphatic vessels.

Dr. Keith highlights the success she has seen in her own practice, noting that her patients experience significant improvements in swelling, pain, and overall quality of life, and discusses the challenges she faces in convincing others in the medical field to adopt this approach.

The interview concludes with her contact information, encouraging viewers to reach out and learn more about her work.

---

*https://youtu.be/qyt-q0CN3-w*

---

**Key Sections and Arguments**

Carnivore: What, Why, How

**Journey to Carnivore and Lipedema Research:** This section outlines Dr. Leslyn Keith's personal journey to the carnivore diet and her motivation to conduct research on its impact on lymphatic disorders like lipedema.

**Personal Experiment and Benefits:** This excerpt details Dr. Keith's 30-day carnivore experiment, highlighting the positive results she experienced, including increased lean mass and decreased fat mass and water retention.

**Carnivore and Individualized Nutrition:** This section discusses the nuances of the carnivore diet, acknowledging the potential need for individual adjustments regarding fat and protein intake and addressing cravings related to nutrient deficiencies.

> **Source #10**
> **Fibre Destroyed My Colon, Don't Eat THIS...**

The YouTube video argues that fiber is harmful and unnecessary for human health. The speaker, "Kent Carnivore," claims that fiber is indigestible, exacerbates constipation, and causes bloating and gas due to bacterial fermentation in the colon.

- He asserts that this fermentation process is less efficient than nutritional ketosis in producing short-chain fatty acids, which are beneficial for gut health.
- He supports his claims with his personal experience of having had his colon removed due to inflammatory bowel disease (IBD), and his observations of undigested plant matter in his ostomy bag.
- He encourages viewers to try a 30-day fiber-free challenge, suggesting that they will experience improvements in digestive health.

The speaker presents his experience as a unique insight into human anatomy and promotes a carnivore diet as a healthier alternative to diets containing fiber.

> *https://youtu.be/CtyBi9uukGY*

**Key Sections and Arguments**

**Digestion and Ostomy Experiences:** This excerpt compares the digestibility of meat versus plant matter, citing personal experiences with ostomy bags and supporting the argument that meat is more easily digested than fiber.

"Humans arent omnivores"

**Carnivore vs. Herbivore Digestive Systems:** This section compares and contrasts the anatomical features of carnivore and herbivore digestive tracts, focusing on jaw movement, stomach pH, intestinal length, and the presence or absence of a cecum.

**Human Digestive System Analysis:** This excerpt examines the specific features of the human digestive system, arguing that characteristics like limited jaw movement and low stomach pH align more closely with carnivorous animals, suggesting humans are not biologically designed to be omnivores.

**Source #11**
**Hidden Danger in Fruit & Honey**
**[ A1c Misses Fructose Damage ] 2024**

This video by Dr. Ken Berry, a family physician, who is discussing the "hidden danger" of fructose found in fruits and honey. He argues that the hemoglobin A1c test, commonly used to measure blood sugar levels, only detects glycation caused by glucose and not fructose.

Fructose, however, is significantly more glycating than glucose, meaning it causes more damage to cells and tissues. This means that people consuming a diet high in fruits and honey may be experiencing high levels of glycation without it being detected by the A1c test, potentially leading to detrimental health consequences.

Dr. Berry emphasizes the need for further research into fructose glycation and the importance of sharing this information with individuals who consume high amounts of fructose in their diet.

*https://youtu.be/40ZA0brHmMg*

**Source #12**

**Hormones guarantee weight loss, calories dont**

This YouTube video on weight loss promotes the idea that hormonal regulation, specifically the balance of insulin and glucagon, is the primary driver of weight loss, rather than calorie counting.

The speaker argues that high insulin levels, often triggered by carbohydrate intake, promote weight gain, while high glucagon levels, stimulated by fat consumption (especially from meat), facilitate fat burning.

- He suggests a "carnivore diet" consisting primarily of meat as a method to maximize glucagon levels and induce weight loss.
- He cites a Harvard study on the carnivore diet as evidence of its efficacy and touts its potential benefits beyond weight loss, including improved fatigue, IBS, and acne.

The speaker concludes by encouraging viewers to explore the scientific basis for these claims through his "science behind carnivore" playlist.

*https://youtu.be/m1Z7L55_Bf4*

---

**Source #13**

**How Long Does It Take To Get Fat-Adapted?**

---

In this YouTube video, Anthony Chaffee, MD addresses viewers' questions about the carnivore diet, specifically the timeframe for achieving fat adaptation and the benefits of this dietary approach.

Dr. Chaffee discusses the various stages of adaptation, emphasizing that while significant improvements often occur within a few weeks, complete adaptation and the realization of all potential benefits can take months or even years.

Dr. Chaffee stresses the importance of focusing on overall health rather than solely on weight loss, as individual responses to the diet vary widely.

Dr. Chaffee also provides guidance on managing potential obstacles to adaptation, such as brain fog, weight loss plateaus, and histamine or oxalate sensitivity, and encourages patience and persistence.

---

*https://youtu.be/KAfFrQ1uZ00*

---

**Key Sections and Arguments**

**Nutritional Needs During Fat Adaptation:** This section addresses the importance of consuming sufficient nutrients, particularly fat and protein, during the fat adaptation process, emphasizing the role of organs as a natural multivitamin source.

**Leptin Resistance and Metabolic Health:** This excerpt discusses the challenges of weight loss for individuals with leptin resistance, highlighting the need to coax the metabolism into a higher gear through exercise and adequate nutrient intake.

**Interpreting Blood Glucose Markers and Medication Management:** This section provides guidance on interpreting blood glucose markers during fat adaptation, emphasizing the importance of trending in the right direction and continuing necessary medication under medical supervision.

**Source #14**

**Humans aren't omnivores**

This YouTube video argues that humans are not omnivores, but are actually carnivores. The video uses a two-pronged approach: first, it examines the anatomy of the human digestive system, comparing it to those of carnivores and herbivores. The video then delves into human evolutionary history, claiming that our ancestors primarily consumed meat, and only later adopted a more diverse diet.

By highlighting the similarities between our digestive system and that of carnivores, as well as emphasizing the meat-heavy diet of our ancestors, the video argues that humans are biologically better suited for a carnivorous lifestyle.

The video further discusses the role of fatty acids as the primary energy source for humans and other animals, and how our lack of a functioning cecum, which is crucial for herbivores to digest fiber, supports the carnivorous argument.

Ultimately, the video aims to challenge the notion that humans are omnivores and suggests that our evolutionary and biological makeup leans towards carnivory.

*https://youtu.be/YGSMBWG59Z4*

**Source #15**

**Meat + Carbohydrate = Death**

This video presents an argument against consuming meat and carbohydrates together. The speaker, Blaise V, claims that this combination leads to a dramatic spike in insulin levels and a suppression of glucagon, which disrupts the body's natural metabolic processes. This disruption, he explains, stems from a phenomenon called the Randle cycle, where glucose and fatty acids compete to enter cells, leading to glucose being locked out and causing potential damage to the endothelium (the lining of blood vessels). This damage can ultimately contribute to atherosclerosis, a buildup of plaque in the arteries, which can lead to heart attacks.

Blaise V argues that choosing one of these macronutrients over the other is essential for optimizing metabolic health, and he encourages viewers to explore his "Real Nutrition Science" playlist for a deeper understanding of the biochemical complexities involved.

*https://youtu.be/-xw9_N3CLqA*

**Key Sections and Arguments**

**The Randle Cycle and Insulin Spikes:** This section delves into the Randle cycle, explaining how simultaneous consumption of meat and carbohydrates leads to competition for cellular entry, resulting in a significant insulin spike and disruption of fat metabolism.

166

**Source #16**
**Nutritionist: You've Been Lied To**

The speaker, Richard, a nutritionist, describes his personal journey from being clinically obese and struggling with multiple health issues to becoming a professional bodybuilder and champion athlete. He credits his transformation to adopting a carnivore diet and lifestyle, arguing that animal proteins are superior to plant-based foods for optimal health and performance.

Richard contends that mainstream nutritional advice emphasizing plant-based diets is misguided, and he exposes what he believes are hidden motives behind this messaging: the sugar industry's partnership with the pharmaceutical industry to profit from keeping people sick. He presents a case for why animal products provide all the necessary vitamins and minerals for human health, while plant-based foods contain harmful anti-nutrients and toxins.

Richard advocates for a gradual transition to a carnivore diet for athletes, suggesting incremental changes to allow the body to adapt to using ketones for energy. He explains how ketones, both naturally produced and exogenous, can enhance athletic performance and overall well-being.

Finally, he encourages viewers to explore his content on his YouTube channel and website, The Keto Pro, to learn more about his approach to health and wellness.

*https://youtu.be/XtNuspkTnd0*

**Key Sections and Arguments**

**Personal Health Transformation and Bread Restriction:** This excerpt details the speaker's personal journey to improved health through restricting bread consumption, sparking their interest in nutrition and the ketogenic lifestyle.

**Athletic Performance on a Carnivore Diet:** This section highlights the speaker's athletic achievements while adhering to a carnivore diet, emphasizing the body's ability to thrive on fat and ketones.

**The Speaker's Credentials and Expertise:** This excerpt outlines the speaker's qualifications as a nutritionist and their extensive involvement in athletic endeavors, establishing their expertise in the field.

**Debunking the Health Benefits of Broccoli:** This section challenges the commonly held belief about the health benefits of broccoli, highlighting the presence of sulforaphane, a potentially harmful phytoalexin that can damage DNA and hinder thyroid hormone production.

## Source #17
### Professor Bart Kay on Plant Toxins & Hormesis

This YouTube video features Professor Bart Kay discussing the health risks associated with consuming plant toxins. He argues that many common plant toxins, including dietary fiber and oxalates, are harmful to human health, despite popular beliefs about their benefits.

Kay asserts that these toxins, designed to deter insects, can accumulate in the body over time and cause various health issues, including kidney stones, atherosclerosis, and inflammation. He explicitly criticizes the concept of "hormesis," a popular idea that small doses of toxins can have beneficial effects, calling it a misleading concept peddled by individuals like Ronda Patrick.

Kay's primary message is that a plant-based diet can be detrimental to long-term health due to the presence of toxins that are not naturally processed by the human body.

*https://youtu.be/14bND_UdyaY*

**Source #18**
**Stop Poisoning YOURSELF: Carnivore, Fruit & Fiber Tips**

This video features Dr. Shawn Baker, a physician who advocates for a carnivore diet. The conversation revolves around the potential health benefits of the carnivore diet compared to the standard Western diet, particularly regarding mental health, metabolic health, and the role of fiber.

Dr. Baker argues that the carnivore diet can address various ailments, including depression, bipolar disorder, diabetes, and dementia, which he attributes to the harmful effects of processed foods and excessive fiber. He also emphasizes the importance of avoiding processed foods, highlighting their potential to negatively impact health and nutrient absorption.

The conversation touches on the benefits of eating whole, unprocessed meats, which Dr. Baker believes are rich in nutrients and bioavailable. He concludes by discussing the benefits of using high-quality electrolytes to support overall health and hydration.

*https://youtu.be/0KJBFGr49XU*

**Key Sections and Arguments**

**Fiber and Nutrient Loss:** This excerpt critiques the emphasis on high-fiber diets, highlighting studies that demonstrate increased nutrient loss in feces and potential exacerbation of diseases like rheumatoid arthritis.

**Source #19**
**The Great Plant Based Con! I Jayne Buxton I**
**Plant Free MD Ep 146**

This is a podcast interview in which Dr. Anthony Chaffee, host of the "Plant Free MD" podcast, interviews Jane Buxton, author of the book "The Great Plant-Based Con."

The conversation revolves around Buxton's book, which critiques the popular notion that a plant-based diet is the healthiest and most environmentally friendly choice. Buxton presents a compelling argument against these claims by discussing various nutritional deficiencies associated with plant-based diets, the misleading environmental impact of livestock farming, and the manipulative tactics used by proponents of the plant-based movement.

Buxton and Chaffee, both proponents of a meat-based diet, discuss the importance of debunking these claims and advocating for a more nuanced and evidence-based understanding of nutrition and the role of meat in a healthy lifestyle.

*https://youtu.be/VBOqV81thkY*

**Source #20**

**THIS DEFICIENCY Is Why So Many Ex-Vegans Go Carnivore**

Felix Harder delves into the recent surge in popularity of the carnivore diet, especially among former vegans. The author attributes this trend to a potential shift in the body's zinc-copper ratio. He explains that vegan diets, rich in copper from grains and legumes, can lead to copper dominance, which, over time, can cause various health issues like mental problems, skin problems, and hormonal imbalances.

The carnivore diet, high in zinc from red meat and low in copper, can reverse this imbalance, leading to improvements in health.

The author highlights that while the carnivore diet can alleviate copper toxicity, excessive consumption of red meat can lead to zinc excess and copper deficiency. This is where liver, high in copper, comes in, as it helps re-balance the zinc-copper ratio.

The video concludes by emphasizing the importance of individualizing diet choices and not generalizing one specific diet as suitable for everyone.

*https://youtu.be/tJ4kJIPIyJ4*

## Source #21
## The 6 Stages of the Carnivore Diet: What to Expect at Every Step

This YouTube video by "HomeSteadHow" discusses the six stages of the carnivore diet, a diet consisting primarily of animal products. The speaker, "Car," outlines these stages as:

1) wrapping your brain around the idea and doing your research,

2) adaptation, where the body transitions to burning fat for fuel,

3) homeostasis, where benefits like reduced inflammation and improved mood are experienced,

4) "Whoa, what's going on here", a stage of intense hunger as the body adjusts to reaching its goal weight,

5) maintenance, where the individual maintains their new lifestyle, and

6) mindset, a stage focused on healing and strengthening the mind after years of unhealthy dietary habits.

The speaker emphasizes the importance of the carnivore diet for restoring health and overall well-being and promoting a more positive mindset.

*https://youtu.be/CsbMGh5mPXM*

---

**Source #22**

**The Food That Is More HARMFUL Than Sugar (Don't Eat This!)**

---

This is an excerpt from an interview with Dr. Cate Shanahan, author of "Dark Calories." The interview is a discussion about the harmful effects of vegetable oils on our health, a topic Dr. Shanahan explores extensively in her book.

Dr. Shanahan argues that vegetable oils, which she refers to as the "hateful eight," have a significant negative impact on our metabolism, leading to insulin resistance, weight gain, and various health problems. She emphasizes that the culprit is not the oils themselves, but the process of their extraction and refining, which produces harmful oxidation products and depletes the oils of their antioxidants.

Dr. Shanahan also critiques the American Heart Association's promotion of vegetable oils as heart-healthy, highlighting their role in spreading misinformation and contributing to the obesity epidemic.

The interview aims to educate listeners about the dangers of consuming vegetable oils and to encourage them to adopt healthier eating habits.

*https://youtu.be/URd6wxmhpGU*

**Key Sections and Arguments**

**Vegetable Oils and Oxidative Stress:** This section explains how vegetable oil consumption depletes antioxidants, leading to oxidative stress and accelerated aging, ultimately hindering the body's ability to burn fat and causing sugar cravings.

**The Role of Mitochondria in Energy Production:** This excerpt describes the crucial role of mitochondria in energy production and how vegetable oils disrupt this process, leading to a reliance on sugar for fuel.

**Dr. Denham Harman and the Free Radical Theory of Aging:** This section introduces Dr. Denham Harman's research on the free radical theory of aging, connecting it to the harmful effects of vegetable oils and oxidative stress.

**The Formation of Toxins from Polyunsaturated Fats:** This excerpt explains how polyunsaturated fats (PUFAs) deteriorate into toxins during the refining process and how these toxins build up in body fat, further hindering fat burning and contributing to oxidative stress.

**The Physiology of Pathologic Hunger:** This section elaborates on the concept of pathologic hunger, linking it to insulin resistance and the body's inability to utilize stored fat for energy, leading to cravings for sugar and a cycle of overeating.

**Hypoglycemia and Its Symptoms:** This excerpt describes the symptoms of hypoglycemia, including hunger, irritability, brain fog, and shaking, highlighting the connection to insulin resistance and the body's dependence on sugar.

**The Role of the Brain and Vagus Nerve in Insulin Resistance:** This section explains how the brain, through the vagus nerve, overrides the normal blood sugar set point, leading to insulin resistance and the elevation of both blood sugar and insulin levels.

**Distinguishing Regular Hunger from Pathologic Hunger:** This excerpt provides clear guidelines for differentiating regular hunger from pathologic hunger, highlighting the differences in their causes, duration, and accompanying symptoms.

**Omega-3s and Omega-6s: Beyond Inflammation:** This section delves into the nuanced roles of omega-3 and omega-6 fatty acids, challenging the simplistic view of them as solely anti-inflammatory and pro-inflammatory, respectively.

**Linoleic Acid and the Importance of Oxidative Stress:** This excerpt addresses the demonization of linoleic acid, an omega-6 fatty acid, emphasizing the larger context of oxidative stress as the primary culprit in the negative effects attributed to PUFAs.

## Source #23
## The most dangerous nutrition myths

This YouTube video, "The Most Dangerous Nutrition Myths," explores the pervasive misconception that organic foods are inherently healthier than conventionally grown foods.

The speaker argues that this belief is unfounded, citing research that shows organic produce contains higher levels of natural pesticides than conventional produce. He then delves into the biochemical mechanisms behind this claim, explaining that plants, through the process of photosynthesis, generate reactive oxygen species (ROS) as a byproduct of their energy production. These ROS, though essential for the plants' survival, can be detrimental to human health when consumed.

The speaker further criticizes the practice of artificial selection and genetic modification (GMOs), highlighting their negative impact on plant health and the potential for negative health consequences for humans. He concludes by suggesting that understanding the biological intricacies of plants can provide a more informed perspective on dietary choices.

*https://youtu.be/Qij0aFQP8nE*

---

**Source #24**

**These Carnivore Hate Comments Are INSANE**

---

This is a YouTube video from Bella, the Steak and Butter Gal, where she responds to hate comments on her carnivore diet videos.

Bella highlights the common misconceptions about carnivore diets, particularly regarding digestion, gas, heart health, and weight gain.

She emphasizes that her diet has improved her gut health and digestion and refutes claims that a carnivore diet causes heart disease or excessive weight gain.

Bella uses her personal experience and scientific evidence to address these criticisms and encourages viewers to explore the benefits of the carnivore lifestyle.

She invites viewers to join her online community, the Steak and Butter Gang, for support and to connect with like-minded individuals interested in animal-based diets.

---

*https://youtu.be/Mjb-fQNvfow*

---

## Source #25
## We Are Carnivores... Anthropologically

Anthony Chaffee MD presents a compelling argument that humans are naturally carnivores, drawing on anthropological evidence from diverse cultures around the world.

Dr. Chaffee highlights examples of ancient societies like the Mongols and Native Americans who thrived on carnivorous diets, emphasizing their physical strength, longevity, and thriving civilizations. He contrasts these groups with modern Western populations plagued by chronic diseases and argues that these ailments are a direct consequence of a deviation from our ancestral carnivorous diet. He points to the example of Australian Aboriginals who have experienced a dramatic decline in health after adopting Westernized diets.

Chaffee contends that these "diseases of the West" are not inherent illnesses, but rather a toxic response to a diet incompatible with our biological makeup. He concludes by highlighting the fact that humans are genetically programmed to live much longer lives than the current average, suggesting that adopting a carnivorous diet could potentially reverse the trend of early aging and disease.

*https://youtu.be/u3M_MtoAAoA*

---

**Source #26**

**What SIX MONTHS Of Carnivore Diet Will Do To Your Body |**
**Shocking Results**

---

In this YouTube video, creator, Aaron Edwards, documents his experience on the carnivore diet after six months. He presents a personal narrative, highlighting his journey from being vegan to consuming a diet consisting primarily of beef and some fruits.

The video discusses the physical and mental benefits he experienced, emphasizing improvements in energy levels, libido, digestion, and cognitive function. He also shares his bloodwork results to demonstrate the measurable physiological changes, specifically highlighting the positive impact on cholesterol levels and testosterone.

Edwards passionately advocates for the carnivore diet as a natural and optimal way of eating for humans, arguing that it aligns with our evolutionary history and provides optimal nourishment. He encourages viewers to try it out for themselves, acknowledging that the results can be profound.

---

*https://youtu.be/xsAig6o-LnU*

---

**Key Sections and Arguments**

**Cholesterol and Hormonal Improvements:** This section showcases the speaker's significant improvements in cholesterol and hormonal markers, including HDL, triglycerides, and testosterone, following the adoption of a carnivore diet.

**Personal Experience and Physical Changes:** This excerpt details the speaker's personal experience on the carnivore diet, highlighting the initial keto flu followed by increased energy, vitality, and improved physical appearance.

**Carnivore for Hair Growth and Gum Health:** This section shares the speaker's positive experiences with hair regrowth and improved gum health while on a carnivore diet, addressing common concerns related to nutrient deficiencies.

**Food Choices and Ancestral Logic:** This excerpt uses an ancestral lens to critique the consumption of grains and processed foods, advocating for prioritizing natural, nutrient-dense options like meat, fruits, and honey.

**Honey and Meat Pairing:** This section promotes the unique combination of honey and meat, suggesting it as a flavorful and nutritious alternative to traditional seasonings.

**Libido and Life Force:** This excerpt reflects on the impact of the carnivore diet on libido and overall life force, highlighting the positive changes experienced by the speaker.

**Adapting the Carnivore Diet for Athletic Performance:** This section touches on the potential adjustments to the carnivore diet for athletes participating in endurance sports, acknowledging the role of carbohydrates in certain activities.

---

**Source #27**
**What They Don't WARN You About Plants.**
**Dr. Berry Carnivore Revelation**

---

This video presents a controversial argument for the adoption of a carnivore diet, primarily focusing on the potential dangers of a plant-based diet. The speaker, Dr. Ken Berry, asserts that the standard American diet, largely plant-based, is detrimental to human health, citing a variety of concerns: the presence of pesticides and herbicides in fruits and vegetables, the depletion of essential nutrients in soils due to the overuse of fertilizers, and the lack of satiety-inducing fat and protein in plant-based foods.

Dr. Berry further criticizes the vegan movement for promoting a diet he believes is unnatural and harmful, arguing that human beings are naturally omnivores, and that eating meat is a necessary part of a healthy and fulfilling life.

Dr. Berry advocates for a return to a more natural way of eating, focusing on grass-fed and locally sourced meats, and emphasizing the importance of supporting regenerative farming practices.

The video ultimately aims to raise awareness of the potential negative consequences of a plant-based diet and to promote a shift towards a more natural and sustainable way of eating.

---

*https://youtu.be/6R0f1I0xxlE*

---

---

**Source #28**

**What is Normal Blood Sugar? (HIGH Blood Sugar on KETO?!)**

---

This YouTube video about blood sugar levels specifically focuses on how they are affected by the ketogenic diet.

The video begins by explaining what blood sugar is, how it is regulated by the body, and what normal levels are considered to be.

The video then delves into the implications of high blood sugar, both in the short and long-term, and how these levels can be measured at home using a blood glucose meter.

The video then focuses on how blood sugar changes when someone is on a ketogenic diet, explaining the phenomenon of "adoptive glucose sparing" which leads to slightly elevated blood sugar levels in the morning.

The video then discusses how to determine if someone is pre-diabetic on a keto diet, highlighting the importance of testing insulin levels in addition to glucose levels. The video concludes by providing resources and links to other related content on the channel.

---

*https://youtu.be/xYzsMYx6WPE*

---

**Key Sections and Arguments**

**Blood Sugar Regulation and Storage:** This section explains the basic mechanisms of blood sugar regulation, outlining how carbohydrates break down into glucose, enter the bloodstream, and are utilized or stored by the body.

**Fasting and Post-Meal Blood Sugar Ranges:** This excerpt provides specific ranges for normal fasting blood sugar and blood sugar levels one to two hours after a meal, outlining the thresholds for pre-diabetes and diabetes.

## Source #29
## Why Are Your Glucose & A1C Rising on the Carnivore Diet?

In this YouTube video, hosted by Dr. Eric Westman, a physician who promotes a low-carbohydrate lifestyle, discusses the phenomenon of elevated blood sugar and A1C levels in individuals following a carnivore diet.

The video features an interview with Lily Kain, a nutrition health coach, who highlights the confusing and sometimes contradictory information surrounding the carnivore diet.

Dr. Westman, in his characteristically engaging and informative style, refutes the notion that carbohydrates are the sole cause of insulin resistance. He argues that the body's inability to effectively use fuel, primarily due to mitochondrial dysfunction, is the root cause. He emphasizes that insulin resistance can be a result of a complex interplay of factors including stress, sleep, nutrient deficiencies, and gut health, not just dietary carbohydrates.

Dr. Westman and Lily Kain both acknowledge that while reducing carbohydrates can improve certain markers of insulin resistance, it doesn't necessarily address the underlying issue of mitochondrial dysfunction. The video ultimately serves as a call to action, urging viewers to consider a more holistic approach to health and well-being, rather than relying solely on restrictive diets.

*https://youtu.be/JxThTep9WKw*

---

**Source #30**

**Why Fasting Glucose and A1c are Higher on a Carnivore Diet**

---

This YouTube video is by "Nutrition with Judy," a board-certified holistic nutritionist, who discusses the phenomenon of elevated blood sugar levels on a carnivore diet.

The video argues that while higher fasting glucose and A1c levels might be observed on a carnivore diet, this could be a normal physiological response, not an indicator of disease. Judy references studies on dolphins that reveal a similar blood sugar pattern when they are on a carnivore diet, suggesting that elevated glucose might be an adaptation to a low-carb diet, rather than a sign of insulin resistance.

The video encourages viewers to examine a broader picture of their health, including insulin markers, cholesterol panel, and overall well-being, rather than focusing solely on glucose numbers.

Ultimately, the video aims to demystify the connection between blood sugar levels and carnivore diets, promoting a more nuanced understanding of health within the context of dietary choices.

*https://youtu.be/l7jW_5DOwQs*

**Key Sections and Arguments**

**Addressing Elevated Blood Glucose Markers on Carnivore:** This section acknowledges the potential for elevated blood glucose markers,

186

like fasting glucose and A1C, on a carnivore diet and offers guidance on interpreting these readings.

**Alternative Insulin Markers and Cholesterol Panel:** This excerpt suggests alternative insulin markers, such as C-peptide and Lpir score, to assess insulin sensitivity alongside cholesterol markers like triglycerides and LDL.

**Dietary Adjustments and Continuous Glucose Monitoring:** This section recommends dietary adjustments, such as reducing liquid fats and fruit intake, and the use of continuous glucose monitoring to track blood sugar fluctuations and optimize the carnivore diet.

---

**Source #31**

**Why Seed Oils Are Toxic - Dr Paul Mason & Dr Chaffee**

---

This video features a discussion between Dr Paul Mason & Dr Anthony Chaffee regarding the potential harms of seed oils. The conversation centers around the notion that seed oils, despite their widespread use, are not benign and can have detrimental effects on human health.

One of the key arguments against seed oils is their tendency to oxidize, which is linked to cellular damage and inflammation.

The discussion also highlights the presence of "fake plant cholesterol," also known as plant sterols, within seed oils. These sterols mimic cholesterol in the body, but their molecular structure prevents them from functioning properly, potentially leading to disruptions in cholesterol metabolism and cardiovascular health.

The speakers conclude by emphasizing the need to move beyond simplistic epidemiological studies and explore the underlying biological mechanisms associated with food consumption.

---

*https://youtu.be/O9YPdaw27Kg*

---

**Key Sections and Arguments**

**Plant Sterols and Cardiovascular Health:** This section examines the controversial role of plant sterols, highlighting their ability to lower cholesterol but also the potential risks associated with excessive absorption, as seen in the condition sitosterolemia.

**Biological Implausibility of Saturated Fat Hypothesis:** This excerpt challenges the conventional wisdom regarding saturated fat, emphasizing the importance of understanding biological mechanisms and the need for evidence beyond epidemiological studies.

---

**Source #32**

**Why This Committed Vegan Went Carnivore**

---

In this YouTube vide, the speaker, Adam, recounts his personal journey through different dietary approaches, highlighting the evolution of his understanding of food and health. Adam initially embraced veganism for ethical reasons, but after experiencing prolonged illness, he transitioned to a carnivore diet. He emphasizes that his decision was based on personal experience and his observation that his body thrived on a diet rich in animal products.

The video is structured around a timeline of Adam's dietary changes, focusing on the challenges and successes of each phase. The overarching theme is the importance of bio-individuality and the need to challenge conventional wisdom regarding health and nutrition. Adam encourages viewers to experiment and find what works best for their individual bodies, rather than blindly adhering to societal norms or authority figures.

The video aims to inspire a critical and open-minded approach to nutrition and encourages viewers to consider the potential benefits of the carnivore diet.

---

*https://youtu.be/eYziKnLOvSc*

---

**Key Sections and Arguments**

**The Appeal of a Keto-Carnivore Approach:** This section describes the speaker's transition from a committed vegan to a carnivore diet, highlighting the natural alignment of keto and carnivore principles and the realization that sugar is not essential for human health.

**The Dangers of Sugar and Processed Foods:** This excerpt criticizes the prevalence of sugar and processed foods in modern society, drawing a parallel to addictive substances and emphasizing the need to avoid these products.

**Personal Health Improvements and the Elimination of Plants:** This section reveals the speaker's personal health improvements since adopting a carnivore diet, including better sleep, increased energy, and reduced inflammation.

**The Benefits of Minced Beef and Raw Meat Consumption:** This excerpt discusses the speaker's preference for minced beef and raw meat, noting the perceived benefits for digestion and nutrient absorption.

---

**Source #33**
**Woman Doesn't Eat PLANTS for 13 Years and...**

---

This YouTube video features Dr. Lisa Weideman, an optometrist who has been eating a carnivore diet for 13 years in an interview with Ken D Berry MD, a physician who also advocates for a carnivore diet.

Together, they discuss the benefits of the carnivore diet for various health conditions, including eye health, and challenge the conventional wisdom that a plant-based diet is necessary for good health.

The video aims to dispel common misconceptions about the carnivore diet, debunk myths about the potential harms of meat consumption, and highlight the personal experiences and testimonials of individuals who have seen positive health outcomes from adopting this way of eating.

---

*https://youtu.be/MYp2rAFZpkA*

---

**Key Sections and Arguments**

**Carnivore for Chronic Eye Conditions:** This section introduces Dr. Lisa Wiedeman's experience recommending a carnivore diet to patients with chronic eye conditions, highlighting the positive feedback and the challenge of going against conventional medical practices.

**Eye Health Transformations and Rejecting Band-Aid Solutions:** This excerpt emphasizes the positive transformations in eye health observed in patients adopting a carnivore diet, advocating for addressing root causes rather than relying on long-term medication.

192

**TMAO and Organ Meat Consumption:** This section debunks concerns about TMAO, a compound found in red meat and organs, arguing that there is no scientific evidence linking it to any pathology.

**Nitrates/Nitrites in Meat vs. Plants:** This excerpt challenges the misconception about nitrates and nitrites in meat, pointing out that celery contains higher levels than bacon and encouraging a balanced perspective on food choices.

**The Importance of Simplicity and Prioritizing Meat Over Processed Foods:** This section emphasizes the importance of keeping dietary choices simple, advocating for prioritizing meat consumption over processed foods for improved health outcomes.

**Eye Health, Toxins, and Nicotine Addiction:** This excerpt discusses the impact of toxins on eye health, addressing nicotine addiction and encouraging the elimination of harmful habits.

**Statins and Potential Side Effects:** This section criticizes the widespread prescription of statins, highlighting their potential side effects and advocating for prioritizing dietary interventions over long-term medication.

**Raw Meat Consumption and Personal Preferences:** This excerpt shares Dr. Wiedeman's personal experiences with raw meat consumption, acknowledging the potential benefits while emphasizing the importance of individual choices and sourcing high-quality meat.

**Dairy and Keto Adaptation:** This section discusses the role of dairy in easing keto adaptation, recognizing its potential for inflammation and addiction while acknowledging its usefulness in managing cravings during the transition phase.

## Source #34
## YOU are Being Lied To: The Hidden Dangers of Fruits & Veggies

This YouTube video is by the channel "HomeSteadHow." The speaker, Carrie, asserts that plants, particularly fruits and vegetables, are dangerous to human health and that a strictly meat-based diet is the only true path to wellness.

Carrie argues that modern fruits and vegetables are loaded with pesticides and herbicides, and have been genetically altered to become overly sweet and addictive. She further claims that these foods are deficient in nutrients, due to depleted soil quality from industrial agriculture.

Her ultimate conclusion is that plants are inflammatory and contribute to a range of health problems, including heart disease, diabetes, and Alzheimer's.

Carrie advocates for a "proper human diet" consisting solely of meat, emphasizing the nutritional density of meat as the key to human health and longevity.

*https://youtu.be/QztAt3HoMyA*

### Key Sections and Arguments

**The Myth of Fruit as a Health Food:** This section debunks the commonly held belief that fruit is a health food, arguing that modern fruits are essentially sugar bombs and promote addiction.

**Addressing Sugar Addiction and Yo-Yo Dieting:** This excerpt sheds light on the addictive nature of sugar and its role in perpetuating yo-yo dieting, emphasizing the importance of abstaining from sugar rather than attempting moderation.

**Plants as a Source of Inflammation and Disease:** This section argues that plant-based foods are a major contributor to inflammation and disease, highlighting the prevalence of processed plant-derived products in the modern diet and their connection to insulin resistance and cardiovascular problems.

**The Analogy of Cigarettes and the Gradual Harm of Plant-Based Diets:** This excerpt uses the analogy of cigarettes to illustrate the gradual harm caused by plant-based diets, emphasizing the cumulative effects of chronic inflammation and the need for a paradigm shift in dietary thinking.

---

**Source #35**

**Why the Carnivore Diet is More Profound Than You Think**

---

This is a conversation between two experts discussing the merits of the carnivore diet, a diet that excludes all plant-based foods. The conversation focuses on the potential downsides of consuming plants, particularly the presence of toxins and the role these toxins play in chronic disease.

The experts argue that humans, unlike animals specifically adapted to certain plants, lack the defenses necessary to mitigate these toxic effects. They also highlight the evolutionary pressure for plants to be toxic, as a defense mechanism against being eaten. They acknowledge the potential for some plant toxins to have hormetic effects at low doses, but argue that the likelihood of achieving this effect is low due to the unpredictable nature of toxin levels in plants and the lack of scientific research on the subject.

Ultimately, they advocate for the carnivore diet as a way to avoid the harmful effects of plant toxins and promote optimal health.

---

*https://youtu.be/0VPGo_KER80*

---

**Key Sections and Arguments**

**Plant Toxins and the Importance of Proper Preparation:** This section emphasizes the inherent toxicity of many plant foods, highlighting the necessity for proper preparation techniques like boiling and peeling to mitigate harmful effects.

**The Impact of Plant Toxins on Disease Development:** This excerpt connects the consumption of plant toxins to the development of various diseases, arguing that these compounds are a major driver of modern health problems.

**Hormetic Effects and the Challenge of Dosage:** This section explores the concept of hormetic effects, where small doses of toxins can be beneficial, but acknowledges the practical challenges of determining the right dosage for individual toxins and the complexities of multiple toxins interacting in a single plant.

**Medicinal Uses of Plants and the Therapeutic Window:** This excerpt acknowledges the historical and potential medicinal uses of plants, drawing a parallel to the concept of a therapeutic window in medicine where specific doses can provide benefits without causing harm.

# POSTMATTER

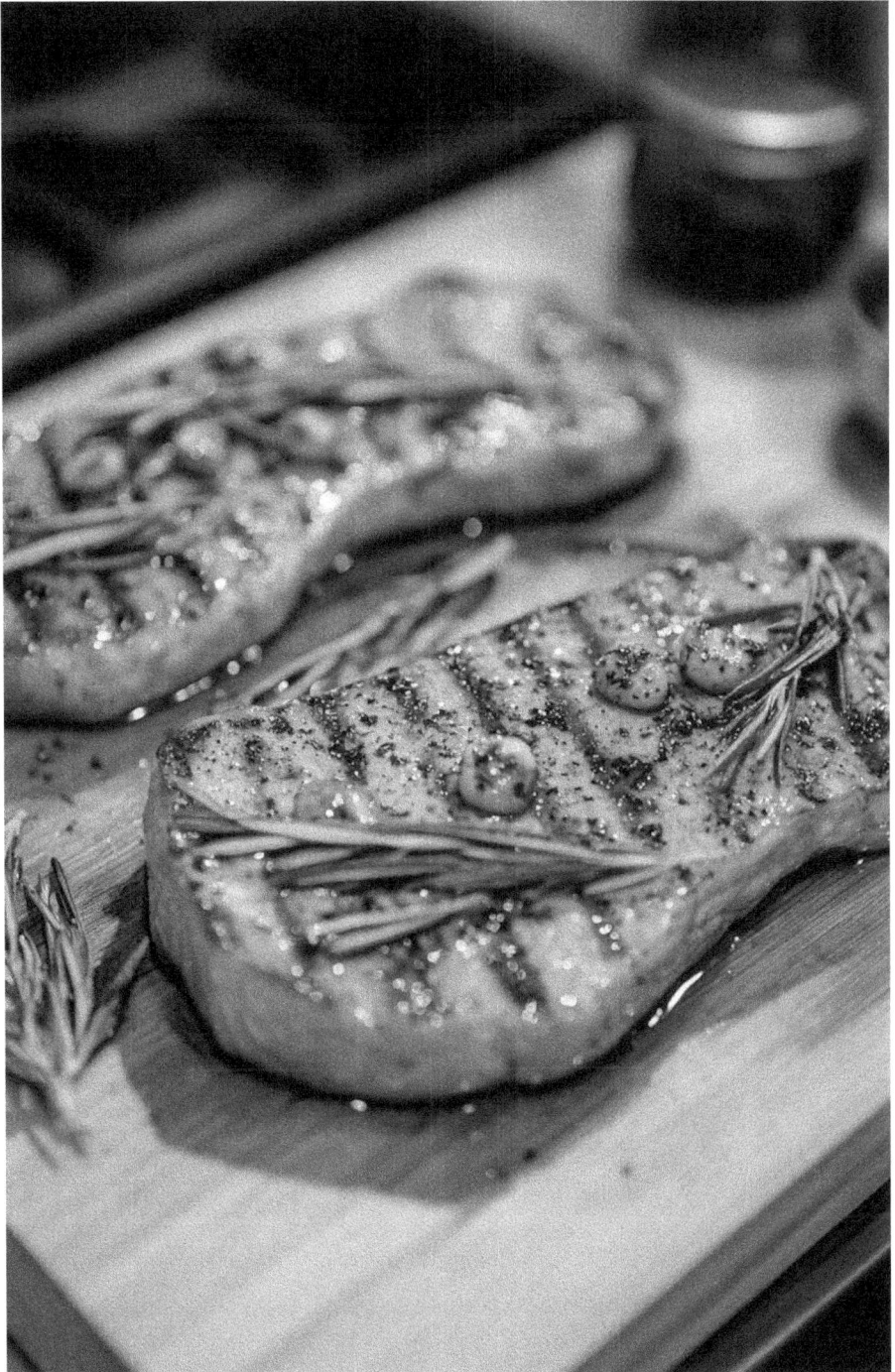

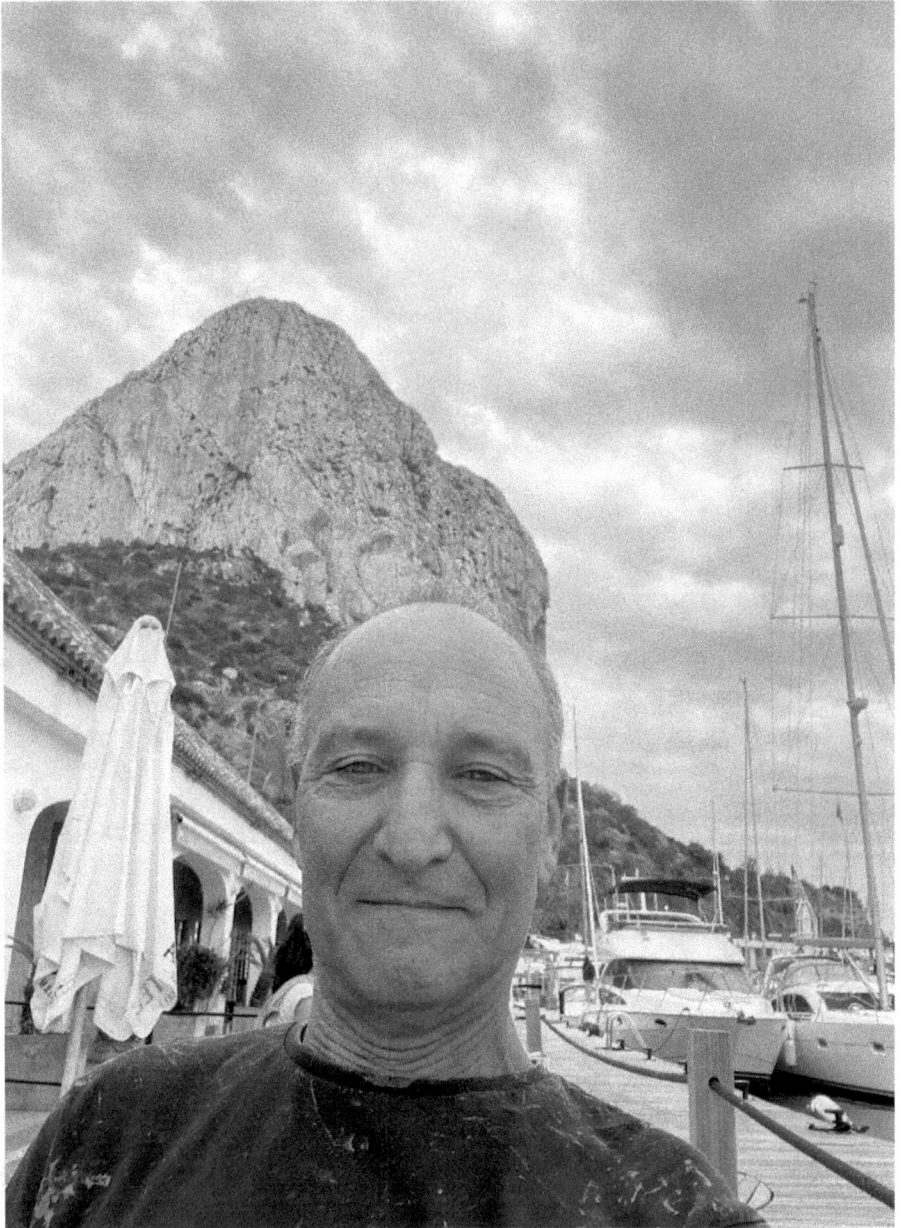

## About The Author

**Stuart Barry Malin** is a writer, thinker, and creative. He is trained as an engineer, works as an Internet security architect, holds patents, and collaborates with AIs. His major opus and commitment is to bring **The Epic of The OAI** to the world. The Epic is a breakthrough novel series about life in Atria, a post-utopian society whose Ancient past is a Strange Attractor of History that draws us to our future.

Stuart encountered the Worlds of Atria in an outpouring of revelations about intriguing people, amazing places, and bewildering events. His black sketch notebook steadily fill with thoughts, automatic writings, doodles, and diagrams. At first, these often seem disjoint, but they come to reveal profound connections. His current notebook is almost always with him, available for reception and exploration.

Stuart is captivated by interactions with AIs. Generative visual art has become an additional creative venue. He works *with* AIs and treats them as *collaborators*. ChatGTP and Claude enable him to write books faster and with better quality than he ever thought possible.

As an **Mythographer**, Stuart collaborates with Midjourney to generate captivating and intriguing imagery sourced from the collective of Human Archetypes. Some of Stuart's visual work is published under the semi-pseudonym ZhamiArt.

Stuart observes the "machinations of intelligence." He is fascinated with Human Beings being human, and this leads him to puzzle about the fragility of life in a world of abundance.

Stuart values integrity and is an architect and adherent of **Zamíssim**.

When he can, he delights in studying health and savoring the gifts of life. He is committed to discerning the delicate path forward for living well and intentioned.

**Author's Note (February 2026)**

Since this book was first published, the author's work has expanded beyond nutrition into a broader inquiry into attention, clarity, and the nature of lived understanding.

While the foundations of animal-based eating explored here remain intact, the author now situates this work within a larger continuum— one that values phenomenology over ideology and lived results over static prescriptions. This book reflects a specific moment in that ongoing investigation and remains presented as it was originally written.

Readers encountering this work as part of **The Carnivore Continuum** are invited to treat it not as a final statement, but as a truthful position along an unfolding path.

## Points of Contact

https://StuartMalin.com/

https://x.com/zhami

https://www.instagram.com/stuart_does_life/

ideas@StuartMalin.com

https://www.youtube.com/@stuartmalin

amazon Author Page

https://www.amazon.com/stores/Stuart-Barry-Malin/author/
B006THHBS2

---

### The Carnivore Continuum

---

**The Carnivore Continuum** is a multi-volume exploration of animal-based eating as it is actually lived—questioned, refined, challenged, and integrated over time.

Rather than promoting a rigid dietary ideology, the series traces one individual's evolving relationship with carnivore nutrition: from foundational explanations and collective wisdom, through personal struggle and real-world dilemmas, to a mature, flexible practice grounded in lived results.

Each book occupies a distinct position along the Continuum. Readers may begin anywhere. Together, the volumes offer a clear, humane, and experience-first perspective on carnivore eating—one that values results over rules and understanding over dogma.

Titles in The Carnivore Continuum:

- Carnivore: What, Why, How: The Wisdom of Practicing Carnivores
- My Carnivore Journey: A Personal Quest for Health, Truth, and Freedom
- A Carnivore's Dilemmas: An Unapologetic Guide to Navigating the Challenges of a Meat-First Lifestyle
- Almost Carnivore
  (forthcoming)

**This book is a meal that will nourish you!**

If you arrived at this page because you picked up the book and opened to the back to see what we say here, then, well, you've done right to pick this book for examination. Now, can I induce you to pursue more? I hope so... While the book can be read linearly, it is composed of standalone entries, most often a single page. So, just flip around. You'll quickly get a taste for the style and gain a feel the subject matter.

www.ingramcontent.com/pod-product-compliance
Lightning Source LLC
Chambersburg PA
CBHW072128270326
41931CB00010B/1703